Intermittent Fasting for Women over 50

A Comprehensive Guide to Understanding IF for Women above the Age of 50 with Recipes

KEITH MALCOM

Contents

Introduction

Intermittent fasting has the benefits like weight loss, mental clarity, a good night's sleep, and a lot more energy. And the first thing was that the belly fat had drastically decreased. Since you can't spot-reduce fat on your body, the loss of belly fat would have been due to hormones, and as it is a known fact that weight gain around the midsection is a part of life during menopause. Post-menopausal are common in women in their 50s, and fat deposition in the waist rises. Belly fat is not only the most difficult to shed, but it is also linked to several health complications, including type 2 diabetes, elevated blood pressure, and heart disease. Intermittent fasting is an excellent way to stay fit and stable when avoiding those problems. Intermittent fasting has been shown in many trials to be particularly effective in lowering belly fat. This is due to a rise in the intake of growth hormone, which aids the body in fat burning.

Intermittent fasting is a calorie restriction method that involves a collection of on and off cycles of feeding. It sounds boring and easy, but it is ensured that it is a self-discipline practice that can be exhausting at first. Intermittent fasting does not alter your eating habits; rather, it alters the timing of your meals. When it comes to losing weight, women over 50 will have a difficult time. A variety of factors can cause this. The most common cause is a slowing metabolism. The higher your metabolism is, the more muscle mass you get.

Intermittent fasting produced less muscle failure than constant calorie restriction, according to a review report. When it is said and done, intermittent fasting can be a very effective weight-loss strategy. Intermittent fasting allows you to consume fewer calories while marginally increasing your metabolism. It's a powerful tool for losing weight and belly fat. Intermittent fasting allows you to eat whatever you want. According to research, fasting has increased appetite and mental wellbeing and potentially deter certain cancers. It will also protect women over 50 from some muscle and joint disorders.

Advantages of Intermitting fasting for women over 50 are:

- Increased energy levels

- Loss of size and body fat

- Increased fat-burning ability.

- Reduced insulin and sugar levels in the blood

- Mental focus and concentration may increase

- Increased energy is a possibility

- Increased growth hormone is a possibility, at least for the short term.

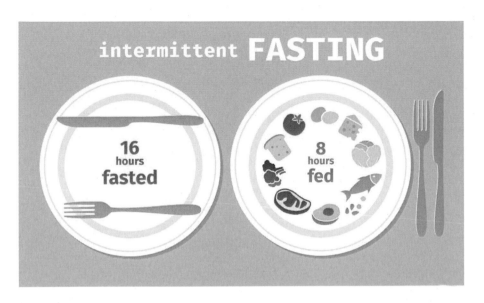

There's also some science at work here, in the form of your body's HGH development. Our bodies generate insulin to accumulate glucose from carbohydrates for future use when we feed. We live in a community where most of our diets are routine, and we are continually bombarded with high sugar and fat foods, which means still gaining weight. Food glucose is processed as fat, resulting in weight gain. Intermittent fasting effectively reverses this process, allowing our cells to use the glucose that has been processed in our cells for energy. Weight loss occurs as cells reach a catabolic (breaking down) state. HGH is activated in response to the body's need for glucose, but when we eat regularly, our HGH output is suppressed because glucose is obtaining from outside sources. HGH is a hormone that regulates metabolism and has many benefits for muscle recovery and fat burning. Fasting for short periods has been shown to increase HGH output by up to 5 times.

Chapter 1: What is intermittent fasting?

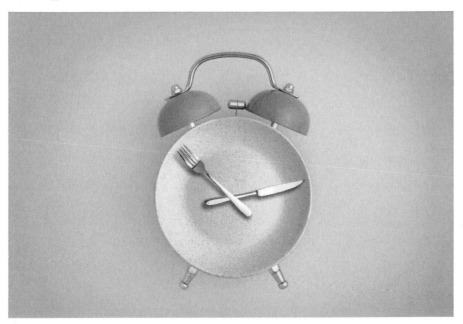

Intermittent fasting has increased in recent years since many people find them simpler to stick to than conventional calorie restriction regimes. If you think about it, IF makes a lot of sense. Notably, since it takes relatively little behavior adjustment, intermittent fasting is one of the best methods for losing weight while maintaining a healthy weight. This is a positive thing as it means IF falls under the category of "easy at doing, but significant enough to make an impact." Enzymes in our gut start to break down we digest, which then become molecules in our bloodstream. Sugar and processed grains are easily destroyed into sugar, which our cells use as energy. If our bodies don't need it all, it's stored as fat. Sugar, on the other hand, can only reach our cells by insulin. Insulin transports sugar into fat cells and retains it there.

Our insulin level drops during meals if we don't eat, and our fat cells will release their accumulated sugar to be used. If we allow our insulin levels to drop, we lose weight. The whole point of IF is to cause insulin levels to drop low that fat is burned off. On restriction days, IF entails limiting caloric consumption for 3 - 5 days a week and eating openly on non-restriction days. Alternate day fasting is a form of intermittent fasting that involves switching between a "fast day" that includes 75% energy limitation and a "eat day" that includes an always available diet. Regular 16-hour fasts or fasting for 24 hours twice a week are two popular intermittent fasting practices. Fasting is much more natural than taking 3–4 meals a day. It is also practiced in Islam, Christianity, and Buddhism for spiritual or moral purposes.

Fasting is a method that can never be mistaken for a strict diet. There is also a lot to think about for women over 50 who want to resume intermittent fasting. When you decide to try it, gradually start and pay special attention to your appetite. If you're always hungry over the day or week, it's probably easier to get back towards a more normal eating routine. Keeping an eye out for signs like nausea, appetite, and low energy. During the day, you should be fueled, energized, and fulfilled, not lethargic and starving.

1.1 How Does Intermittent Fasting Work?

You won't have to deprive yourself if you practice intermittent fasting, also known as IF. It also doesn't permit you to eat a lot of unhealthy food when you aren't fasting. Rather than eating snacks and meals during the day, you feed over a fixed period.

The majority of people adhere to an IF schedule that allows them to fast for 12 to 16 hours every day. They eat regular meals and snacks the majority of the time. Since most people sleep for around eight hours during their fasting hours, committing to this diet plan isn't as difficult as it sounds. You're also advised to drink zero-calorie beverages like water, coffee, and tea.

For optimal intermittent fasting results, build an eating routine that works for you. Consider the following example:

• **12-hour fasts:** A 12-hour fast entails skipping breakfast and waiting until lunch to eat. You might eat an early supper and skip evening snacks if you want to have your morning meal. A 12-12 fast is reasonably easy to manage for most older women.

• **16-hour fasts:** A 16-8 IF plan will help you achieve faster results. Within 8 hours, most people prefer to eat two proper meals and a snack or two. For example, the eating window may be set during noon and 8 p.m., or between 8 a.m. and 4 p.m.

- **5-2 routine:** You might not be able to stick to a restricted eating schedule every day. Another choice is to follow a 12- or 16-hour fast for five days and then relax for two days. For example, you might do intermittent fasting throughout the week and feel full on the weekends.

- **Alternate-day fasts:** Another choice is to eat very few calories on alternate days. For instance, you might restrict your calories to under 500 calories per day and usually eat the next. It's worth noting that regular IF fasts never necessitate calorie restrictions that low.

You'll get a great outcome from this diet if you stick to it. At the same time, on special occasions, you should take a break from this sort of eating routine. You should try various forms of intermittent fasting to see which one fits better for you. Many people begin their IF journey with the 12-12 plan and then move to the 16-8 plan. After that, try to stick to your schedule as closely as possible.

1.2 What Makes Intermittent Fasting Work?

Some people claim that IF has helped them lose weight simply because the small eating window forces them to eat fewer calories. For example, instead of three meals and two snacks, they can only have two meals and one snack. They become more conscious of the foods they eat and avoid refined carbohydrates, unhealthy fats, and empty calories.

Of course, you have the freedom to eat whatever healthy foods you choose. While some people use intermittent fasting to minimize their total calorie consumption, some use it in conjunction with a keto, vegan, or another diet.

Women's Intermittent Fasting Benefits Could Go Beyond Calorie Restrictions

Although some nutritionists believe that IF only succeeds because it encourages people to eat less, others disagree. They assume that intermittent fasting produces better results than traditional meal schedules with the same number of calories and other nutrients. Studies have also proposed that fasting over many hours a day accomplishes more than just calorie restriction.

These are some of the metabolic changes which IF induces that can help explain the synergistic effects:

• **Insulin:** Lower insulin levels during the fasting cycle will aid fat burning.

• **Human Growth Hormone (HGH):** As insulin levels fall, HGH levels increase, encouraging fat loss and muscle growth.

• **Noradrenaline:** When your stomach is empty, your nervous system sends this chemical to your cells to tell them they ought to unleash fat for food.

How much time will our body take to adjust?

Intermittent fasting takes 2 to 4 weeks for the body to become familiar with it. When you are becoming used to the new schedule, you might crave sugar or be irritable. However, researchers observed that test subjects who make it past the transition process are more likely to adhere to the schedule and feel better. Water and zero-calorie drinks like black coffee and tea are allowed on days when you are not consuming "regularly eating" during your cycles do not imply "going insane." If you fill your meals with fast food, fried foods, and desserts, you are not losing weight or getting healthy.

What does it do for the human body?

Intermittent fasting does more than burning fat.

- Usually, prolonged fasting improves working memory and verbal memory.

- It can help with blood pressure, resting heartbeats, and other cardio metrics.

- A research was conducted where a group of people who fasted for 16 hours lost weight while retaining muscle mass.

- While in another research, it was found that overweight adult humans lost some weight by prolonged fasting in six small trials.

- Intermittent fasting is found to minimize tissue injury.

1.3 Is Intermittent Fasting Healthy?

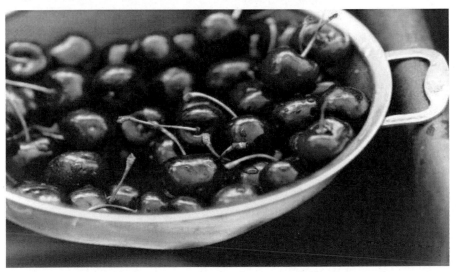

Is intermittent fasting a healthy way to eat? Remember that you can only fast for 12 -16 hours at a time, not for days. You still have A LOT of time to eat a delicious and nutritious meal. Of course, few older women may require regular eating due to metabolic disorders or medication instructions. In any case, you can speak to your doctor about your eating habits before making any adjustments.

Although it isn't fasting, some doctors say that allowing easy-to-digest foods like whole fruits during the fasted state has medical benefits. Modifications like these will also provide a much-needed break for your digestive and metabolic systems. For example, the famous weight-loss book "Fit for Life" recommended consuming fruit after supper but before lunch.

Despite not adhering to the diets other guidelines or counting calories, PEOPLE lost weight and improved their health. This plan may have succeeded precisely because dieters substituted junk food for whole foods. In either case, participants considered this dietary adjustment to be beneficial and simple to implement. Traditionalists won't call this fasting, but it's good to realize that you have choices if you can't go without food for more than a few hours.

1.4 Typical Intermittent Fasting Results

In the medical literature, a chiropractor Dr. Becky, and ABOVE -50 HEALTH coach, says it's difficult to find any drawbacks to IF. She clarified that the blood sugar and insulin would drop to dangerously low levels during the fasting phase. Your body will depend on stored fat for energy if insulin's hormonal fat-storing signaling is not present.

The National Library of Medicine has also released an analysis of women's health-related sporadic fast outcomes. Research on the IMPLEMENTATION of fasting as a method to minimize the risk of DIABETES, cancer, and other metabolic disorders, as well as heart disease, are among the report's highlights.

1.5 Is Intermittent Fasting the Best Fat-Loss Tool for You?

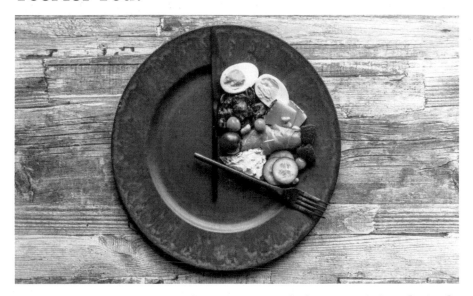

In any case, IF seems to function greatly because it is relatively simple to follow. By reducing eating windows, people claim it helps them naturally reduce calories and make healthier food choices. According to some research, IF tends to encourage fat loss while sparing lean muscle mass, making it a better choice than simply reducing calories, carbs, or fat.

Of course, the majority of people combine IF with yet another weight-loss technique. To lose weight, you might try and eat 1,200 calories per day. It could be better to spread 1,200 calories over two meals and two snacks rather than three meals and three snacks. If you've had difficulty losing weight because your diet didn't work or was too difficult to follow, you may want to try intermittent fasting.

Dr. Kathryn Waldrep suggests eating within 8 hours and selecting the period depending on the body's circadian cycles in Prime Women's newly launched plate weight loss program. Eat during 9 a.m. and 5 p.m. if you're an early riser. Night owls will eat their first meal around noon and their last meal around 8:00 p.m. There tends to be reliable data on the validity of this method to eat for weight loss as further research on IF and circadian cycles are performed.

Before incorporating these ideas into your lifestyle, consult your doctor, as you would, for any dietary adjustments. This knowledge is given solely for educational reasons and does not constitute medical advice.

1.6 Intermittent fasting Has 10 Proven Health Benefits

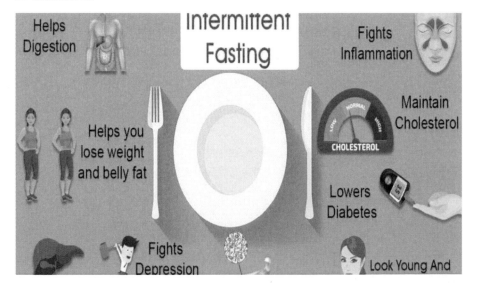

IF is an eating practice in which you switch between eating and fasting times. Intermittent fasting can be achieved in a variety of ways, like the 16/8 or 5:2 routines. Numerous studies have shown it can have important health and cognitive benefits. Here are ten health advantages of intermittent fasting that have been scientifically proven.

1. Intermittent Fasting Changes The Function of Cells, Genes, and Hormones

When you don't eat for a while, your body goes through several changes.

To make stored body fat more available, your body, for example, initiates essential cellular repair processes and adjusts hormone levels.

Here are some of the physiological changes that happen during fasting:

• Insulin levels: Insulin levels in the blood drop dramatically, promoting fat burning.

• Human growth hormone: Growth hormone levels in the blood will rise by up to 5-fold. Increased levels of this hormone aid with fat loss and muscle growth, among other things.

• Cellular repair: The body initiates essential cellular repair procedures, such as removing waste from cells.

• Gene expression: There are beneficial variations in various genes and molecules connected to survival and disease prevention.

These variations in hormones, gene expression, and cell function are linked to several advantages of intermittent fasting.

Insulin levels fall, and human growth hormone levels rise when you fast. Your cells also initiate critical cellular repair processes and alter the expression of genes.

2. Intermittent Fasting Can Help You Lose Weight and Belly Fat

Many people who experiment with intermittent fasting do so in terms of weight loss. In general, intermittent fasting causes you to eat fewer meals. You will consume fewer calories unless you compensate by consuming even more often during the other meals.

Intermittent fasting also improves hormone function, which aids weight loss. Reduced insulin levels, greater growth hormone levels, and higher norepinephrine levels help the body break down fat and use it for energy.

As a result, short-term fasting boosts metabolic rate by 3.7-14%, allowing you to eat even more calories. Intermittent fasting, in other words, operates on both ends of the calorie equation. It increases your metabolic rate (calories expended) while decreasing the quantity of food you consume (reduces calories).

According to the scientific literature 2014 review, intermittent fasting results in a weight loss of 3 to 8 percent over 3 to 24 weeks. This is a huge number. The participants also lost 4 to 7 percent of the waist circumference, showing they lost excess belly fat, the disease-causing fat in the abdominal cavity.

3. Intermittent fasting will lower the risk of Type 2 diabetes by reducing insulin resistance.

In recent decades, type 2 diabetes is becoming extremely popular. The high blood sugar level in the sense of insulin resistance is the most prominent characteristic. Anything that decreases insulin resistance and protects against type 2 diabetes should decrease blood sugar levels.

Intermittent fasting has tangible advantages for insulin resistance and results in a significant drop in blood sugar levels. Intermittent fasting has been shown to lower fasting blood sugar by 3-6 percent and fasting insulin by 20-31 percent in human studies.

Intermittent fasting also prevented diabetic rats from kidney injury, which is one of the most serious complications of diabetes. This means that intermittent fasting could be very beneficial for people at risk for type 2 diabetes.

There might, however, be some gender differences. According to a study, after a 22-day intermittent fasting regimen, blood sugar control in women worsened. At least in men, intermittent fasting can lower insulin resistance and lower blood sugar levels.

4. Intermittent fasting can help the body decrease oxidative stress and inflammation.

One of the steps toward aging and many chronic diseases is oxidative stress. It includes unstable molecules known as free radicals interacting with and destroying other essential molecules (such as protein and DNA). Intermittent fasting has been shown in many studies to improve the body's resistance to oxidative stress.

In addition, studies show that intermittent fasting can help tackle inflammation, which is a major cause of a variety of diseases. This should help prevent aging and the onset of a variety of diseases.

5. Intermittent fasting may be good for your heart.

Heart disease is still the world's leading cause of death. Various health indicators (also known as "risk factors") have been linked to a decreased or increased risk of heart disease.

Intermittent fasting has been shown to increase blood pressure, inflammatory markers, blood triglycerides, blood sugar levels, and total and LDL cholesterol, among other risk factors.

However, a significant portion of this is focused on animal research. Before any recommendations can be made, further research on the impact on humans' heart health is needed.

6. Intermittent fasting activates several cellular repair mechanisms

When we fast, our bodies' cells start a process called autophagy, a cellular "waste removal" process. Broken and damaged proteins that accumulate within cells over time are broken down and metabolized by the cells. Increased autophagy can protect against cancer and Alzheimer's disease, among other diseases.

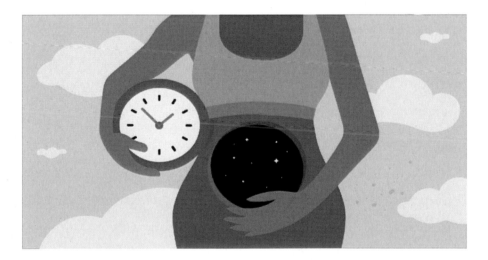

7. Intermittent fasting can aid in cancer prevention.

Cancer is a horrific disease that is characterized by uncontrollable cell development. Fasting has also been shown to have several metabolic benefits, including a lower risk of cancer.

Despite the lack of human studies, promising evidence from animal studies suggests that intermittent fasting may help to hinder cancer. Fasting minimized multiple side effects of chemotherapy in human cancer patients, according to some evidence.

8. Intermittent fasting is beneficial to your mental health.

What is beneficial for health is frequently also good for the brain. Intermittent fasting increases a variety of metabolic characteristics that are related to brain health.

Reduced oxidative stress, blood sugar levels, inflammation, and insulin resistance are all part of this. Intermittent fasting has been shown in many experiments in rats to increase the development of new nerve cells, which could boost brain function.

It also raises brain hormone levels known as a brain-derived neurotrophic factor (BDNF), whose deficiency has been related to depression and other neurological issues. Intermittent fasting has also been shown to protect against brain damage caused by strokes in animals.

9. Intermittent fasting can reduce the risk of Alzheimer's disease.

The most prominent neurodegenerative disease in the world is Alzheimer's disease. Since there is no cure for Alzheimer's disease, stopping it from occurring in the first place is important. According to a rat study, intermittent fasting can delay the onset of Alzheimer's disease or minimize its severity.

According to a series of case reports, a lifestyle modification that included regular short-term fasts substantially boosted Alzheimer's symptoms in 9 out of 10 patients. According to animal studies, fasting may also defend against other neurodegenerative disorders, such as Parkinson's and Huntington's disease. However, further human research is needed.

10. Intermittent fasting can help you live longer by extending your life span

One of the most intriguing benefits of intermittent fasting is the potential to prolong life span. Intermittent fasting increases lifespan in rats in the same way as constant calorie restriction does. The results of a few of these experiments were very dramatic. One of them found that rats who fasted every other day survived 83 percent longer than rats who didn't fast.

Intermittent fasting has become very common among the anti-aging crowd, even though it has yet to be demonstrated in humans. Given the benefits of intermittent fasting for metabolism and various health indicators, it's easy to see how it could assist you in living a healthier and longer life.

1.7 The Drawbacks: Four Intermittent Fasting Side-Effects

So far, intermittent fasting seems to have a positive impact. However, if a diet isn't approached correctly, it can still have a drawback. The following are four possible drawbacks or "cons" of intermittent fasting:

1. Weight Gain Can Still Occur Despite Intermittent Fasting

When you're fasting, you may feel starved, making you more susceptible to binge eating when you're not fasting. You'll gain weight even though you go rogue during your non-fasting times.

And if you fast for 16 hours a day, eating more calories than your body burns can result in a long-term rise in body fat.

Fasting Suggestion

The quality of your food is extremely significant. Plan your meals ahead of time and ensure you eat nutrient-dense foods during your non-fasting times. Every day stay within your daily calorie quota.

Intermittent fasting is not a replacement for balanced eating or calorie restriction. It offers no instructions about what you can eat, which an obvious necessity for good is dieting. Consider it a method that assists us in determining what we should feed.

2. Fasting will make you tired and depressed.

Often People who miss meals complain of exhaustion and mood changes, including irritability. Many people even show poorer cognitive functioning, which they believe affects their ability to work. This tends to be particularly true of people who fast for long periods, such as observing an alternate-day fasting eating schedule.

Fasting Suggestion

For many people, short-term fasting is a healthier alternative. For certain people, missing breakfast and not eating for 12 or even 16 hours may be a more fruitful long-term strategy. If you're going to fast for a long time, pick a day of the week or a period when you won't need to be too busy or concentrated.

3. Meal skipping can result in headaches, dizziness, and nausea.

Fasting for long periods can cause low blood sugar, leaving you feeling dizzy, lightheaded, with headaches and nausea. Fasting for long periods can cause blood glucose levels to drop. Hypoglycemia is a disorder characterized by low blood glucose levels.

Although minor drops in blood glucose can benefit your overall health, they can be harmful or even fatal for people with type 1 diabetes and those taking diabetic drugs. If you have any medical issues, check with your doctor to see if intermittent fasting is safe for you.

4. Restrictive Eating Can Lead to Eating Disorders

Any diet that encourages missing meals or restricting one's food intake can lead to some unhealthy food interactions in some people, particularly when the benefits of not eating are directly affected by not eating whatsoever.

The more you fast, the fewer calories you'll be able to consume and the more weight you'll be able to lose. Some people could be tempted to go too far with intermittent fasting as a result of this. In addition, not getting enough calories per day can cause nutritional deficiencies and eating disorders in some people.

Fasting Suggestion

Make sure you're receiving all of the vitamins you need to keep your body working while you're fasting. Create a meal strategy that fits you with the aid of a dietitian or a doctor.

You may also try intuitive eating, which turns the attention away from calories and determination and toward knowing what your body requires to survive, regardless of the time of day or when your next authorized eating window is.

1.8 Is an Intermittent Fasting Diet Worth Trying?

Intermittent fasting has many possible health benefits, but there isn't enough evidence to tell whether you are doing something to boost your health. Implement basic nutrition concepts that have been well developed by science to improve your health if you chose to pursue intermittent fastings, such as calorie restriction to maintain a healthy weight and a balanced diet that includes all of the necessary micronutrients.

Often consult your doctor or a dietitian before making any significant dietary adjustments to ensure that your new regimen is healthy for you.

Your diet is more than half the fight, whether you're pursuing intermittent fasting or simply trying to lose weight. Get on track with your balanced diet with portion-controlled, ready-to-eat meals delivered right to your door.

1.9 Is Intermitting Fasting different for women?

Biological gender norms have influenced men and women's hormonal reactions to carbs, lack of sleep, and even fasting. Men and women reacted to times of abundance and shortage distinctly in hunter-gatherer cultures. Fasting resulted in a massive increase in metabolism in men, owing to their greater overall size. This metabolic increase provided them with the energy they needed to hunt. When men have not eaten much, their genetic code says, "Go find food for everybody. "According to research, human evolutionary adaptations to times of shortage can still be found today. Men's metabolisms improve by 14% during brief fasting cycles.

On the other hand, women do not react to intermittent fasting in the same way men do. Women's bodies reacted to times of shortage differently than male bodies in hunter-gatherer cultures. In surviving a long-term drought, women's metabolic rates slowed to save calories and store fat. What this suggests for today's women is that intermittent fasting might be the difference for them. Women are usually advised to fast for just 14–15 hours because they tend to do well with shorter fasts. Many women tend to be healthy by using modified forms of intermittent fasting. On the other hand, various studies have found that fasting days can cause hunger, mood fluctuations, loss of focus, decreased stamina, nausea, and bad breath. According to some reports on the internet, women's menstrual cycles have also been said to have ceased while on an intermittent fasting diet.

1.10 Is intermittent fasting safe for women over 50?

Females may benefit from intermittent fasting in particular. Since a female body has a greater percentage of fat than a man's, intermittent fasting seems to be an ideal option for women who are obese or want to lose weight more quickly. When striving to lose weight, the body will burn out food and starch reserves within about 8 -10 hours after feeding and only begins to burn fat for strength. Intermittent fasting could be the solution for women trying to shed weight despite maintaining a balanced diet and fitness schedule.

1.11 Who should not try intermittent fasting?

Many individuals use intermittent fasting to lose fat, while others use it to treat medical conditions, including inflammatory bowel disease, elevated cholesterol, etc. Intermittent fasting, on the other hand, is not for all. Before you try intermittent fasting or some other diet, make an appointment with your physician. Few people who should avoid experimenting with intermittent fasting:

- Those who have had an eating disorder in the past.

- Those who have diabetes

- Have some blood sugar issues.

- Are underweight.

- On medications.

- Have low blood pressure.

Individuals who are not in these groups and can easily go for intermittent fasting can go forever. It can become a lifestyle improvement with several advantages. Intermittent fasting can have various consequences depending on the individual, and it is not meant for everybody. If you have fatigue, discomfort, or other symptoms after beginning intermittent fasting, see your doctor.

Chapter 2: Methods of intermitt fasting

There are different types of IF to pick from. Choose the kind that best suits your lifestyle, and then discuss it with your doctor.

2.1   16/8

The method is used daily. This is the most often used IF form. A 16/8 is commonly used in the regular system. This entails consuming normal, nutritious meals for six to eight hours per day and then fasting for the next 16 to 18 hours. This has been discovered to be the most long-term form. You can eat 2-3 meals during the feeding time. Fitness gurus have popularized this form, which is also very easy to follow. It is as basic as not eating something after dinner and missing breakfast to follow this fasting process. If you have your last food at 8 p.m. but do not eat again until noon, you will have fasted for 16 hours. Others like to feed about 9 a.m. and 5 p.m., allowing plenty of time for a nutritious breakfast at 9 a.m., a regular lunch at midday, and a light evening meal or snack at 4 p.m. while you begin your fast.

You should experiment to find the Period that works best for you. It is important to focus on consuming nutritious foods during your eating window. If you eat a lot of fast food or consume an unhealthy number of calories, this approach would

to provide a selection of nutritious whole
al, such as:

, apples, berries, peaches, oranges, pears, and

Vegetables: Broccoli, cucumbers, cauliflower, leafy greens, onions, and other vegetables

Whole grain: Quinoa, rice, beans, barley, buckwheat, and other whole grains

Protein: Legumes, nuts, meat, eggs, poultry, fish, grains, and other sources of protein

However, when fasting, sugar drinks such as water, coffee, and unsweetened tea will greatly reduce your hunger while leaving you hydrated. Eating sweets or going overboard on sugary snacks, on either hand, may counteract the benefits of 16/8 and could end up causing more damage than good to overall health. It is easy to implement, adaptable, and long-term viable.

Advantages

Saves time and money: It is also useful because it will help you save time and money you spent cooking and food preparation. Not only does limiting your diet to several hours each day help you shed calories during the day, but tests indicate that fasting will also improve your appetite and promote weight loss.

Reduces insulin levels: It's been shown to decrease insulin levels by 34% and blood sugar levels by 4–7%, effectively lowering cholesterol levels. To get started, experiment with different timing options. A 12/12 diet involves feeding for 12 hours and then fasting for 12 hours.

Disadvantages

A problem with skipping breakfast: It helps reduce weight, but so many people cannot skip the first meal of the day.

Not enough calorie restriction: During the eight-hour cycle, you can eat quite enough calories and as many different types of food as you would like. This does not educate you regarding healthier eating and can increase calorie consumption, which is unhealthy and can lead to weight gain.

2.2   Method

This method entails consuming regular, nutritious meals five days a week and restricting oneself to 500-600 calories two days a week. It's uncertain if eating all of your calories in one sitting or spreading them out over the day is better, so do what works for you. It is very easy to describe the 5:2 diet. You eat regularly for five days a week and do not have to worry about calorie restriction. You can cut your calorie consumption to a fifth of your normal requirements on the remaining two days. This equates to around 500 calories a day for women. One can fast every two days of each week you like. Fasting on Mondays and Thursdays with 2 or 3 balanced meals, then eating regularly for the remainder of the week, is a popular form of preparing the week. It is worth noting that eating "normally" does not imply that you can eat whatever you want.

If you eat fast food in excess, you will not lose weight and might even gain weight. You can eat as well as you would if you were not fasting at all. The 5:2 diet's versatility is a big part of its popularity. You won't have to obey any complex menu schedules, and you won't have to weigh servings or carb counting. To encourage fat loss and weight management, you can start consuming healthy foods on every eating schedule. To fill up your stomach on fasting days, continue to consume elevated, low-calorie foods. Carrots and broccoli, which are rich in nutrition, are excellent options for keeping your whole. You can drink whatever you want on normal eating days, but sticking to pure water or low-calorie drinks is the best option on fasting days.

You can try to stretch out the fasting days as far as possible. Eating a lot of high-volume foods can aid. If you are sticking to 500-calories a day, you might eat 200 calories for breakfast, 100 calories for lunch, and 200 calories for dinner. You might still consume 250 calories at brunch and only 250 calories at dinner. This is not easy to go from eating all day properly to just eating 500 calories twice a week. Begin by gradually lowering your calorie intake. Decrease the diet from 2,000 to 1,500 calories

throughout the first week, for instance. Try just 1,0[...]
the following week. Decrease your calorie consumpti[...]
you are taking the 500–600 calories needed on fasting [...]
you have never experienced fasting previously, [...]
remember that there's a fair risk you'll feel adverse effects [...]
fasting days.

Choose your fast days: You will feel more comfortable making healthier decisions if you concentrate on the timing of meals instead of the eating itself. You should select your fasts on the 5:2 diet, depending on your calendar. Most individuals fast during the week because it's easier to stick to a schedule, particularly if you've many social interactions on weekends.

No restriction of foods: Since no meals are legally banned, socializing with others can be simpler. It would also help you feel less hungry on days where you are not fasting.

Health benefits: It has been linked to various health impacts, including losing weight and better blood pressure and heart health.

Cons:

Difficult transition period: While the 5:2 diet can be manageable once you have gotten used to it, it does take some real commitment at first. You will probably experience extreme hunger and other side effects in the first several fasts, including

However, once you've gotten through
...dy can adjust, and you'll feel more

...ten opens up the possibility of
...an this lead to the negative side effects of
...t it can also prevent you from achieving your
...sing weight.

...o calories
...n before
...ays. If
...lease
...on

.3 Stop Eating

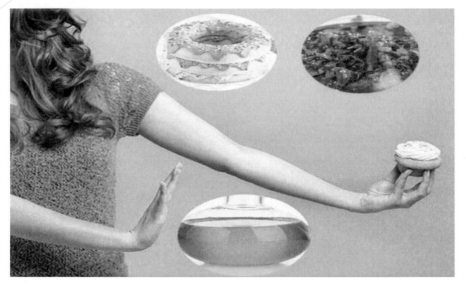

This refers to a perfect 24-hour fast if you fast from dinner one day to dinner the very next day; for instance, you have done a perfect 24-hour fast if you end dinner at 7 p.m. Tuesday but do not eat again until dinner 7 p.m. Wednesday. The outcome is the same if you fast from dinner to dinner or breakfast to breakfast. During the short, liquids such as water and other low-calorie drinks are tolerated, but food items are not. You must diet properly during the feeding cycles while you are trying to lose weight. In other terms, you could eat as much as you would if you were not fasting at all. Since Eat Stop Eat is a form of intermittent fasting, it is designed to function in the same way as anyone else.

It will help you reduce your calorie consumption despite having you think about it too much. When you do not have as much time for lunch as you used to, it is much more difficult to consume the same number of calories in a week. Once you do eat, you will find it hard to overeat since your stomach has reduced slightly due to the fast. Eat Stop Eat can also help to kickstart your metabolism. If you reduce the feeding time, you provide a fasting cycle during which the system must use its own accumulated glycogen from carbs and fats as food, and if those reserves are depleted, the body enters a ketosis and burns fat for energy. If you fast a long time, your body begins fat burning instead of carbohydrates for energy. Eat around 2,000 calories per day for women for the next few days; never fast on days in a row.

After a few days of regular eating, you can fast again and continue the cycle. In any given week, do not fast more than twice. A calorie deficiency of 10% can be achieved by fasting even once a week. You are not required to eat any particular foods, such as carbohydrates; in reality, a limited diet on non-fasting days can reduce your energy. You should eat a variety of citrus, herbs, and spices. 20 to 30 grams of high-quality protein per 4 - 5 hours for a maximum of around 100 grams per day of protein. If required, any of which can be obtained from protein powder. If you notice yourself adding weight between fasts, reduce your food intake by 10% on non-fasting days.

Advantages

More muscle strength: The Eat Stop Eat method is almost as good at losing weight as reducing carbs by a certain percentage per day, and it also helps dieters keep more muscle strength.

Easy to follow: It might be less confusing and transparent than diets that need you to exclude a whole food category, such as fat or carbohydrates.

Disadvantages

Health issues: Few individuals may have headaches and irritability due to the diet, so it is not recommended for individuals with diabetes, pregnant mothers.

Increased cravings: Since you have "saved" calories, the package allows sugary beverages, making you want candy or prefer unhealthy foods.

There is no proper guidance: It makes no clear meal-plan guidelines for non-fasting days, allowing you to exercise incredible self-control and decide what and how to eat for yourself — an environment where many individuals are struggling with their weight need advice.

2.4 Alternate day fasting

Often regarded as every-other-day dieting, switches four days of calorie counting (500 calories for women) with three days of eating openly. Consider it as a cycle of feast and fast so. For alternating-day fast, you shift between feeding and fasting days. Although experts are divided on the effectiveness of this solution to weight loss, the basic concept and promise of the method remain the same. Fasting flips the metabolism turn, so you start eating fat for food rather than the glucose contained in your liver. This promotes weight loss as well as other fitness advantages. Seeking an alternate-day fasting regimen that works for you can be difficult. Fortunately, there are a variety of alternate-day fasting schedules accessible.

You can consume up to 500 calories on fast days and drink plenty of zero-calorie drinks as you want. To feel fuller for longer on fasting days, aim for 50 grams of protein and low-calorie vegetables like a salad with grilled chicken, etc. You should eat anything you like and on feast days. It does not appear to affect what food you eat as long as the overall calorie intake is limited. Many individuals do not overeat on feast days while fasting every other day. On feast days, individuals only consume 10% more carbohydrates than average, according to studies. Alternate-day fasters usually lose 5 to 10 pounds every three months, which is greater than most intermittent fasting methods like time-restricted eating, restricting eating times to a specific time a day.

On the ADF diet, when an individual loses weight, they burn fewer calories. This is not a symptom of hunger but rather a natural adaptation. According to one study, within six months of implementing an ADF schedule, people who are obese lose about 6.8% of their body mass. On the other hand, intermittent fasting may produce comparable weight loss effects as prolonged caloric restriction, according to a 2017 study.

Advantages

Autophagy: This form of fasting can also promote autophagy, a mechanism through which the cells eliminate protein build-up and dead or weakened cell structures.

Decrease in blood pressure: In this type of IF, studies have also shown reductions in **blood pressure** and **insulin resistance**, a precursor to type 2 diabetes that occurs when your body grows resistant to the effects of the hormone insulin.

Disadvantages

Time took: According to a 2017 survey, 15 percent of alternate-day fasters quit, compared with 26 % of daily dieters who limited carbohydrates. Not everybody enjoys calorie counting each day. It requires time to adapt to this feeding method, but in general, alternate-day fasters tend to gain hold of their appetite after about ten days.

2.5 The Warrior Diet Method

Among the first common diets to incorporate a method of intermittent fasting was the Warrior Diet. The Warrior Diet requires people to fast for 20 hours throughout the day and night, then overeat for 4 hours each night. This approach is founded on the assumption that our forefathers lived their lives by hunting during the day and feasted at night. During the fasting period, eat limited amounts of dairy, eggs, and raw vegetables to keep yourself going. Water, green tea are all zero-calorie or low-calorie drinks. To guarantee that you get sufficient basic vitamins and minerals, it is smart to eat a few portions of fruit and vegetables during the day. During the feeding time, there are no limits. Although you might order a burger, it is better to eat balanced, nutritional foods like fruits and vegetables. Throughout your feeding window, whole-grain foods, including sprouted wheat flour, quinoa, and oatmeal, are all excellent choices for refueling. Protein is recommended, and organic and full-fat dairy products; you can also have butter, yogurt, and raw milk.

Like in every diet, you can strive to limit a few foods and drinks, such as those rich in sugar and sodium. You can eat very little carbs over the 20-hour fasting cycle. Whenever it is time for your eating window, you can eat as much as you want before the four hours are up. You can choose your eating window based on whatever timeline fits best for you. However, most people prefer to eat in the evening. When it is time to eat, consider focusing your foods on healthy fats and significant amounts of protein, particularly milk protein sources like cheese and yogurt. The Warrior Diet eliminates the need for carb counting and thus emphasizes whole, unprocessed ingredients. Timing is a crucial aspect of this protocol. Long cycles of fasting and short hours of overeating lead to optimum wellbeing, nutrition, and body structure.

Since the Warrior Diet has no changes once you deviate from the 20:4, you are no longer on the Warrior Diet. There isn't much evidence to back up the effects of this form of fasting; intermittent fasting, in particular, has been related to a variety of beneficial effects, ranging from losing weight to increased brain health. While some individuals may benefit from the Warrior Diet, most will find the guidelines too complex to adhere to, but the Warrior Diet can be beneficial.

Advantages

May aid weight loss: As you are fat for 20 hours, the ketosis will start after 12 hours and help you reduce weight regardless of whether you are eating anything for 4 hours.

May improve blood sugar: It helps in lowering your insulin that improves the blood sugar level.

May help with inflammation: heart disease, asthma, certain tumors, bowel defects, and other diseases caused by inflammation. This form of intermittent fasting, according to research, can help combat chronic inflammation.

Disadvantages

Can lead to overeating: Fasting for 20 hours straight can result in extreme appetite and cravings, which can add to overeating and health issues.

Other health issues: Trying to deprive your body of significant calories will lead to nausea, difficulties concentrating, "hanger," mood fluctuations, depression, anxiety, lightheadedness, hormone disturbances, and other issues.

2.6 Spontaneous meal skipping method

You would not have to stick to a strict intermittent fasting schedule to enjoy any of the advantages. A further choice is to miss meals on occasion, including when you are not hungry or when you are very lazy to prepare and eat. It is a fallacy that people must feed every few hours or risk malnutrition or muscle loss. Your body is designed to withstand long stretches of hunger, much less missing 1 or 2 two meals now and then. As a result, if you are not hungry that day, miss breakfast and enjoy a nutritious lunch and dinner instead. Alternatively, if you are out and can't locate something you want to consume, go on a quick fast. A random spontaneous fast is when you skip either one or two meals when you seem like it.

During the other meals, make sure to eat nutritious snacks. If you wish to try intermittent fasting, remember that the consistency of your food is important. It's impossible to hope to lose weight and improve your fitness by bingeing on fast food at meal times. If you plan to start IF but do not want to leap straight in, meal-skipping is a good option. When you are not hungry, miss the meal next time. You may feel hungry, but it will pass quickly, particularly if you do not concentrate on it. To also have a good evening, work over the lunch break and finish an hour early. If you plan to skip a meal, avoid drinking something with fat content, such as juices or sodas. Instead, when fasting, sticking to low-calorie beverages like coffee, tea, and water is the best option.

Advantages

Flexible: it is one of the easiest types of intermittent fasting, and you do not need to go through the hassle of planning a meal.

Time-saving: you have to select a time for skipping a meal, and that's it.

Disadvantages

Slow weight loss: it is the easiest type of if, but unfortunately, you will see the results very slowly. Usually, you will lose 0.26 pounds in a week and maybe 1 kg in a month.

Does not have a proper guideline: if you are trying to lose weight and are obese

2.7   Lean gains method:

A usual lean gains schedule begins with a one-hour exercise in the middle of the day. At 1 p.m., the exercise will be preceded by the start of the fed state. At 4 p.m., you will have your second meal, and at 9 p.m., you'll have your last meal. This lean gains ritual is famous since most individuals find fasting right after getting up to be easier. Fasting is made easier by the ability to take a cup of breakfast. A lean gains routine from 1 to 9 p.m. sounds like early morning and a late meal. Since it is a personal decision about which portions are larger or equivalent, it might be more prudent to have two larger meals and a smaller meal somewhere between. As a result, at 1 p.m., you would have enough strength to return from the fasting phase, and at 9 p.m., you should have enough energy to finish most of your activities for the fasting period.

It is essential to know that you don't have to follow this exact schedule. Everyone's routines and priorities are different. You can adjust the hours to fit your timetable as long as you're willing to fast for 16 hours. Regardless of the routine you choose, make sure to stick to it. The lean gains plan will be easier to adjust to if you keep a daily eating schedule. Black coffee, tea, and sugar-free gum, etc., are all acceptable within the fasting time because they have no calories. It is okay to apply a bit of milk to your cup, as well as something else that is still under ten calories.

The lean gains usually recommend a routine that replaces macros during the week. The carb and calorie consumption should be maximum on training days, with lesser carbohydrate and higher fat intake on non-training days. It is suggested that your post-workout meal be the biggest meal of the day. During rest periods, your initial meal might be the biggest of the day, responsible for about 40% of your total calorie intake.

Advantages

Flexibility: The simplicity that this method provides is a big explanation for many lean gains' successes. Any intermittent fasting plans call for only one or two big meals during the day. It is fine to be adaptable. Your progress will not be determined whether your initial meal serves 30 percent or 40 percent of your overall daily calories. If you like to eat the biggest meal at night and it reliably helps you achieve your goals, then continue doing what you're doing.

Improved metabolism: Responsive thermogenesis will cause your metabolism to slow down over the years. Short-term fasting, on the other hand, can potentially boost your metabolism. Fasting can also benefit your metabolic health by influencing signaling pathways that boost mitochondrial function, aid DNA repair, and enhance overall metabolic health. Ten. Fasting at night has also been shown to alter the gastrointestinal micro-biota, leading to great metabolic health changes.

Health benefits: Intermittent fasting could combat disease mechanisms by triggering efficient cellular stressors signaling pathways Intermittent fasting has been shown to lower insulin levels by up to 32% and blood sugar levels by 4-6% in studies. As per a 2016 report, the lean gains procedure will result in better biomarkers such as lower insulin and blood glucose levels and lower body fat linked to higher energy consumption.

Disadvantages

Nutrition/Eating disorders: Prolonged fasting can be avoided by someone who suffers from an eating disorder. It is beneficial, but it may become a source of violence for those suffering from an eating disorder.

Stress issues: Individuals with a high propensity to stress must use caution before starting an intermittent fasting regimen.

Counting calories is time-consuming: Most people would not want to waste time measuring and calculating their food.

2.8   Crescendo fasting:

For women, this is one of the easiest and healthiest options. It is one of the most affordable methods for weight loss. It does not necessitate the use of additional instruments such as drugs, nor does it necessitate the use of pricey exercise facilities. What it asks is for strong and serious fasting self-control. The simple approach is to fast for 12 – 16 hours 2-3 times a week on alternating days. The "fasting window" is 12-16 hours, and the "feeding window" is 8-12 hours. This method of fasting is a lot less difficult to adopt. Merely skipping breakfast is a simple way to get started.

You may encounter food cravings at first, but they will pass, and after you have become used to it, appetite will not be an issue. You will expand your fasting window to prolong the fat-burning Period during intermittent fasting while your system tries to adapt and your hormones stay healthy. You will probably understand that when fasting, you concentrate, which is the exact reverse of what you would imagine, but it is something that most individuals feel. It is a gentler way of acclimating the body to fasting. When women fast in this manner, they can lose more weight while still gaining a lot of energy. Crescendo fasting can be performed twice a week on different days. This implies that you just fast 2 or 3 times a week. It is best to stop fasting on successive days. While you fast on Wednesday, for example, the next fasting days must be Friday and Sunday.

Drink lots of water during your fast to stay hydrated. One can also consume coffee, tea and a little bit of milk can be added.

Advantages

Reduces the risk of heart diseases: Intermittent fasting lowers blood sugar, lowers heart disease and stroke risk. In addition, crescendo fasting has been shown to increase blood pressure and reduces the risk factors for cardiac failure and multiple medical conditions.

Benefits brain: Fasting has been shown in several experiments to have profound effects on brain health. Fasting improves concentration and concentrating, response time, instant recall, intelligence, and the development of new neurons, among other neurologic advantages. Fasting has also been shown to decrease inflammation in the brain and aid regeneration post-stroke or brain damage.

Increases weight loss by accelerating metabolism: Often, calorie-restricted diets cause the metabolism to decelerate. Intermittent fasting, on the other hand, has the opposite effect. If we do not eat for a while, our systems will use surplus fat as a source of energy before we feed again. We start burning fat for energy, which promotes weight loss.

Decreases insulin production and the possibility of diabetes: Diabetes is prevalent, and its prevalence is increasing by the day. Diabetes is simply described as a disorder in which the system has an excessive amount of sugar. As a result, cells cannot respond to insulin and will not draw in more and more glucose from the bloodstream. Glucose levels rise as a result of these activities. It can help solve this problem by reducing blood sugar levels, thus reversing insulin sensitivity.

Disadvantages

Might feel dizzy: Your body will take time to adapt to this routine, but while doing so, you might feel dizzy or feel strong cravings.

Can lead to overeating: Fasting for 20 hours straight can result in extreme appetite and cravings, which can add to overeating and health issues.

Chapter No. 3: Intermittent fasting anti-cancer and anti-aging study

Will calorie restriction CR or fasting help the body prevent cancer? May it also aid in the more successful treatment of cancer?

Fasting and CR can help delay or even stop cancer growth, destroy cancer cells, strengthen the immune system, and increase radiation and chemotherapy therapy efficacy.

3.1 What is it?

Table 1. Definitions of Calorie Restriction and Fasting

Term	Definition
Calorie Restriction	For a long period, 20 to 40 percent reduction in calorie intake (1200 calories for women vs. 1400 calories for men per day)
Intermittent Calorie Restriction	For short periods, 50 to 70 percent reduction in calorie intake (600 to 1000 calories per day)

Fasting	For anywhere from 1 day - several weeks, complete avoidance of calorie intake
Intermittent Fasting	Complete avoidance of calorie intake for 16 to 18 hours daily or alternating a fasting day with a normal energy intake day

Fasting is one of medicine's oldest remedies. Fasting has been advocated as an integral method of prevention and healing by many respected doctors throughout history and by many of the traditional healing systems. Fasting, according to Hippocrates, allowed the body to recover itself.

Fasting is practiced in almost every faith culture, including Christianity, Buddhism, Judaism, Hinduism, and Islam. Many of history's great spiritual figures, like Jesus, Buddha, and Mohammed, fasted for spiritual and mental clarification. Mahatma Gandhi, the Indian emperor, fasted for 21 days to foster peace in one of the most well-known political events of the twentieth century.

Humans have experienced many long stretches of famine in history, and while many factors affect this, it seems that most humans can live on water alone for over a month. Many species have evolved to survive in conditions with fluctuating food supply, in which starvation was a common occurrence, and evolution has been chosen for organisms that can tolerate starvation.

3.2 What is the Evidence?

There has been more than a century of research into the function of calorie restriction in the likelihood of living longer. Although most of this research has been conducted on livestock, a small amount of data is collected on humans, suggesting a beneficial effect on secondary aging. In humans, risks for atherosclerosis and diabetes, as well as inflammatory markers like C-reactive protein (CRP) and tumor necrosis factor (TNF), are significantly reduced after CR (Holloszy). We'll be looking into the studies on calorie restriction, fasting, and cancer in particular. We'll start with a glance at the physiological processes being investigated before moving on to some fascinating human studies.

3.3 Biological sciences

To mitigate the harm that would reduce health, an organism must divert energy into several defensive systems to adapt to starvation. According to Drs, these systems can also help extend the life and reduce the risk of cancer. Fontana and Longo of the University of Southern California, CR without deprivation, is the most potent and repeatable physiological intervention for extending lifespan and shielding mammals from cancer. CR decreases levels of anabolic hormones, growth factors, and inflammatory cytokines, lower cell proliferation and oxidative stress increases autophagy (cell death),

Insulin-like growth factor-1 is one of the main metabolic factors listed above (IGF-1). Dr. Longo makes an interesting observation: CR was only effective in lowering IGF-1 when protein intake was also limited. Increased IGF-1 was linked to a high protein intake or a positive nitrogen balance. This is significant because many cancer patients are advised to raise their protein intake through treatment; this advice will need to be reconsidered.

There are several issues with CR. One is to achieve the metabolic changes mentioned above, and it takes weeks, if not months. Another issue is that it usually leads to long-term weight loss. With moderate (20%) CR, a weight loss of at least 15% is predicted. This may be ideal for overweight individuals, but it may result in underweight and malnutrition for those at a healthy weight or who are now at a marginal weight.

Intermittent CR/intermittent fasting is another choice for CR, and it may be more supportive and less troubling for weight loss. It can cause fat storage, IGF-1, and cell proliferation to decrease while rising insulin sensitivity and adiponectin levels. These findings come from the first rodent studies of spontaneous mammary tumor models, in which fasting on alternating days was compared to fasting for 2-3 day periods per week. Both methods decreased tumor incidence by 40-80% relative to ad-lib feeding in various models, but the results were more pronounced with alternate-day intermittent fasting.

During food deprivation or fasting, the body goes through three stages of metabolism. Dr. Longo and Dr. Lee go into greater detail about these. The first step, which can last up to 10 hours, depletes glycogen stores for energy. As glycogen reserves are depleted, the body switches to glycerol and free fatty acids generated from adipose tissue as a source of energy. Ketones are produced by these nutrients, which the brain and body can use for energy. Based on the person's size and health, this process will last many weeks.

As defined in the Low Carbohydrate Diet portion, a ketogenic diet may also move the source of energy from glucose to fatty acids, in addition to fasting. The ketogenic diet can theoretically be maintained longer if calories and other necessary nutrients are ingested, but some patients may find the diet difficult to handle. When fat stores are depleted during fasting, muscle breakdown starts to keep gluconeogenesis going.

Fasting, unlike CR, produces improvements in cellular defense that initially protect against weight loss while also increasing resistance from oxidative stress. Compared to CR, fasting causes a more pronounced decrease in insulin levels and a rise in insulin sensitivity in a brief period. Since insulin levels are linked to cancer risk, these variations may have clinical implications.

Furthermore, cancer cells are thought to be resistant to cancer treatment and the immune system because they do not react to fasting protective signals. Differential stress tolerance is the term for this operation (DSR).

3.4 Research Studies

Carlo Moreschi published the first research paper in 1909, stating that CR prevented the growth of tumors transplanted into mice. Since then, a wide body of research has shown that CR slows tumor growth in various animal models. Extensive studies in both monkeys and rodents have shown that beginning CR at 12 months increases lifespan and decreases random cancers by 50%. While most cancer cells appear susceptible to CR, some cells have mutations that render them immune to the treatment. This means that CR's effectiveness could be restricted to a subset of cancers. Human studies have been limited so far, but there have been some promising results in cancer risk reduction and treatment-related side effects reduction.

3.5 Tumor Regression and Risk Reduction

Longo and colleagues showed in 2014 that fasting triggered "old" immune cells to death in mice, which were substituted by stem cells once the mice resumed feeding. They concluded that a three-day fast could aid in the regeneration of a strong immune system. They also found that a 48-hour fast delayed the growth and spread of five of the eight cancers studied in mice. They found that combining fasting cycles with chemotherapy was more successful than chemotherapy alone in all cancers surveyed. Since these were all animal experiments, it's unclear if humans would benefit in the same way; however, some ongoing clinical trials look into the effects of calorie reduction or fasting against cancer.

A 2007 study (n=16) found that alternate-day fasting, wherein calories were restricted to 400 for women and 600 for men on one day and unrestricted on the other, decreased blood glucose, insulin, and IGF-1 levels, as well as the risk of chronic diseases such as diabetes, cancer, and cardiovascular disease. Studies of two calorie restrictions, one involving women at slightly elevated breast cancer risk (n = 19) and the other involving newly diagnosed pancreatic cancer patients (n = 19), revealed a reduction in serum markers (IGF, fatty acid desaturase, stearoyl-CoA desaturase, and aldolase C), which could be linked to risk of cancer and prognosis.

The new research analyzed data from the Women's Healthy Eating and Living study and discovered that breast cancer survivors who fasted for at least thirteen hours a night had a 36% lower risk of recurrence and a 21% lower risk of breast cancer-related mortality. This discovery's proposed mechanism is linked to improved glycemic regulation, which protects against carcinogenesis. Overnight fasting was related to increasingly lower hemoglobin A1C levels for each 2-hour rise in fasting time. This study is especially intriguing since it focuses on a dietary plan that most people might adopt.

3.6 Protection from Treatment-Related Side Effects

Fasting can also help patients avoid the negative side effects of radiation or chemotherapy. Before treatment, fasting for up to five days followed by a normal diet may minimize side effects without rendering chronic weight loss or interacting with the treatment's therapeutic impact. Patients over the age of 50 (n=10) who voluntarily fasted before and after chemotherapy showed fewer side effects. Compared to chemotherapy without fasting, a small study (n=6) found that fasting decreased fatigue, exhaustion, and gastrointestinal side effects. The majority of participants that always fasted before chemotherapy also showed a pattern for a decrease in several additional side effects, as shown in Figure 2.

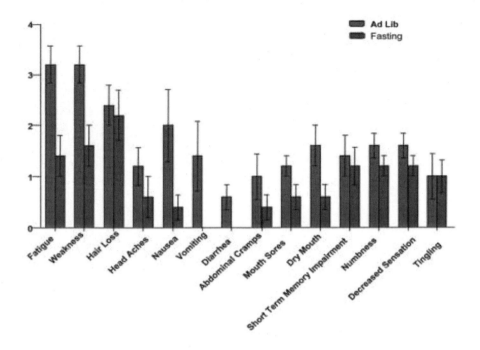

FIGURE: AVERAGE SELF-REPORTED SEVERITY OF SYMPTOMS IN PATIENTS THAT RECEIVED CHEMOTHERAPY WITH OR WITHOUT FASTING

3.7 Safety

Fasting (350 kcal/day) was healthy and helpful to people with chronic diseases (rheumatic diseases, chronic pain syndrome, hypertension, and metabolic syndrome) in a large cohort study of 2000 people. In terms of cancer, the most serious problem with calorie reduction and fasting is weight loss. Weight loss is less of a problem with short-term fasting than with long-term calorie restriction, as previously stated. This may be a beneficial side effect for overweight people; however, for cancer patients who are either underweight or trying to keep their weight, further weight loss can be harmful and make fasting or CR impossible. It's also worth noting that fasting for more than a few days can cause side effects like headaches, light-headedness, fatigue, and nausea. Fasting for several weeks can cause side effects like amenorrhea or anemia. The more difficult it is to re-feed after a long easy, the more crucial it is to be careful. To avoid serious problems–or even death–when coming off a long fast, this step must be incremental and gradual.

3.8 Suggestion

Fasting seems to have more drastic outcomes and defense of healthy cells than CR, without the possibility of losing weight or immune suppression. Both fasting and CR are still being researched, and conclusive findings will have to wait for the results of such studies. It may not be suitable for all, especially those underweight or just very sick, and should never be tried without trained practitioners' guidance, as previously stated.

Here are some takeaways:

1. Eat an anti-inflammatory diet rich in colorful fruits, vegetables, grains, lentils, herbs, and spices in general.

2. Consumption of low- to moderate-carbohydrate foods with low-glycemic starches

3. Eat healthy fats at any meal, like Omega-3 sources.

4. Consume 3-4 ounces of protein per meal from a mixture of plant and animal sources.

5. Increase the time between breakfast and dinner to enable a longer overnight fast, aiming for 13 hours or more. For example, dinner at 6:00 p.m. and breakfast at 7:00 a.m.

6. Short-term water-fasts of 1-3 days to help the immune system regenerate and improve cellular defenses against oxidative stress. You should work with a health professional to decide how often a quick is suitable for you.

7. Water fasting can be considered for cancer patients 2-3 days before treatment and up to one day after treatment to improve treatment effectiveness and minimize treatment-related side effects, but only under a competent practitioner's supervision.

3.9 Is it possible to reverse the effects of aging by intermittent fasting?

Fasting has a wide range of effects on the body. If you don't eat for a longer period, the body will need to find some energy source to keep itself going. It draws on stored fat to meet its energy requirements. However, the body must change its hormone levels to access this fat. All of this triggers changes that can assist turn back the clock:

1. There is an increase in the production of human growth hormones (HGH).

The pituitary gland produces human growth hormones. This hormone is involved in a variety of bodily functions. HGH is needed for the following functions:

- Muscle growth

- Cell repair

- Exercise performance

- Metabolic rate

- Strength

Unfortunately, as people get older, their HGH levels drop. This is true for people and pets. HGH levels in humans are thought to decrease by 14-15 percent per ten years after 20-30. As a result, by the time you reach 60, the HGH levels are usually half of what they've been at 25.

Low levels of HGH may have a detrimental impact on health and well-being and hasten the aging process. According to a 1990 study, age-related HGH decline can lead to a loss of lean body mass and a rise in fat tissue mass. HGH also appears to help with rehabilitation following an illness or injury, according to research. Intermittent fasting has been shown in studies to be a natural way to increase HGH yield. As a result, IF can be beneficial in reversing a few of the effects of aging.

2. Cells also have a chance to repair themselves

The body's resources and energy can be depleted by digestion. When the body is allowed to have free time from digestion, such as by fasting, it has the opportunity to focus on cellular repair. Autophagy is one of the most important aspects of the repair process. The term "autophagy" refers to the act of consuming oneself. That is an accurate summary of what happens during this phase.

The body's cleaning processes kill old cell membranes that have accumulated over time as autophagy occurs. These old membranes can harm the performance of cells. The body's HGH sends out a signal to generate replacements as they are removed. Autophagy assists the body in recycling and renewing its cells in this way. According to research, autophagy is induced by intermittent fasting; consequently, IF plays a critical role in kicking off a phase that can eventually reverse aging.

3. Gene expression that prolongs life is supported.

Your genes will express themselves completely differently from IF. This move will help your nervous system live longer and protect your neurons from genetic and environmental influences that can harm them as you get older. Defending the nervous system in this manner will aid in brain aging performance. As a result, IF can play a role in lowering your risk of age-related neurodegenerative disorders like Alzheimer's disease.

3.10 Anti-cancer and Anti-aging effects

Central obesity, insulin resistance, high blood pressure, and dyslipidemia are all signs of metabolic syndrome. Metabolic syndrome is a major risk factor for several cancers. A pilot study in 14 metabolic syndrome patients who fasted (no eating or drinking) from sunrise to sunset for more than 14 hours daily for four weeks was conducted to see if intermittent fasting from sunup to sundown had an anti-cancer effect.

This pilot study has significant clinical implications, especially in intermittent fasting to prevent cancer in people with metabolic syndrome. Regular intermittent fasting can be divided into two types depending on when it begins: fasting begins at sunrise and ends at sunset (dusk). The fasting begins at a self-determined time of day and lasts for a fixed number of hours, including both human activity (daytime) and inactivity (nighttime) periods; Fasting that begins at a self-determined time of day and lasts for a fixed number of hours, including both human activity and inactivity periods

Ramadan fasting is a unique type of intermittent fasting that occurs from dawn to dusk without eating and drinking during the lunar calendar month of Ramadan and has many distinct characteristics: Fasting occurs exclusively during human daytime hours from dawn to dusk and includes both eating and drinking, which distinguishes it from the dawn to dusk intermittent fasting. This fasting pattern is thought to allow energy reserves to be accessed without causing micronutrient deficiencies resulting from replenishment after sunset.

Fasting during the day's active hours tends to be important for cancer prevention and care. A study found that mice who did not have access to food during the operation phase of a 12-hour light/12-hour dark period had significantly slower tumor progression, and survival than mice who did not have access to nutrition during the sleepiness phase had free access to food. The mice without any access to food, mostly during the activity, had the best anti-cancer response, while those with unrestricted access to food had the worst outcome. In mice without any access to food, mostly during inactivity, there was a small anti-cancer effect but no survival benefit. In humans, a study of 2413 people with breast cancer who did not have diabetes mellitus found that fasting for 13 hours or more at night was related to a lower risk of breast cancer recurrence. It's worth remembering that there were no control subjects in this study who only fasted during the operation hours.

For four weeks, intermittent fasting from sunup to sundown induces main insulin signaling regulatory proteins and increases insulin resistance.

At the end of the fourth week of intermittent fasting, key regulatory proteins of insulin signaling, including VPS8,

POLRMT, and IGFBP5, were induced, as was PRKCSH one week after the fourth-week intermittent fasting. During 4-week intermittent fasting, the induction of VPS8, POLRMT, and IGFBP5 GPs at the end of the fourth week followed the substantial decrease in insulin resistance measured by HOMA-IR one week later. VPS8, a subunit of the CORVET complex, is involved in integrin-dependent cell adhesion and migration and beta-1 integrin recycling. Integrins are transmembrane receptors that bind the extracellular matrix to the cell's actin cytoskeleton, acting as a cell adhesion sensor. Insulin resistance can be caused by impaired integrin signaling in the extracellular matrix of skeletal muscle, adipose tissue, and the liver. Insulin synthesis requires healthy skeletal muscle and beta-cell mitochondrial function. Skeletal muscle mitochondrial dysfunction and decreased oxidative ability are linked to type 2 diabetes mellitus. POLRMT is a gene that codes for mitochondrial RNA polymerase, which is involved in pancreatic beta-cell transcription and insulin secretion69. Since the loss of POLRMT causes significant mitochondrial dysfunction in cardiac muscle, the loss or dysfunction of POLRMT in beta-cells should cause similar mitochondrial dysfunction, resulting in insulin resistance and diabetes mellitus

Chapter No. 4: Best Food and types of Intermittent Fasting

Intermittent fasting has risen to the top of the list of diets for women over 50. It's also the foundation of PLATE, our weight-loss program. It also doesn't need costly cookbooks, time-consuming manuals, or even a specialized trainer or dietician, ALONG WITH its anti-aging and weight-loss results. However, it's also important to note that the foods you consume while intermittently fasting are just as important as the timing of the fast. Continue reading to discover the best foods to consume for intermittent fasting to maintain better health and weight loss.

First and foremost—Make a schedule for your intermittent fasting.

PLATE, a weight-loss program, suggests the 16:8 Intermittent Fasting schedule because it works better for women. However, since everybody is different, you might find that a different schedule is more appropriate. Before learning more about the healthiest meals for intermittent fasting, take a look at these other fasting schedules:

- ADF or Alternate Day Fasting: One day of ad libitum eating is followed by one day of full fasting.

- ADF or Adjusted Alternate Day Fasting: One day of usual feeding accompanied by a very low-calorie diet (about 25% of normal caloric intake).

- 2/5: Two days of complete fasting followed by five days of ad libitum eating.

- 1/6: Complete Fasting for one day of the week, then eating normally the rest of the week.

- TRF or Time Restricting Feeding: Fasting for 12-20 hours a day (as a continuation of the nighttime fast) with a "feeding window" of 4-12 hours on each day of the week. This is where our PLATE app fits in.

Here are the best foods to consume during intermittent fasting, now that we've explained the fasting schedules and time windows.

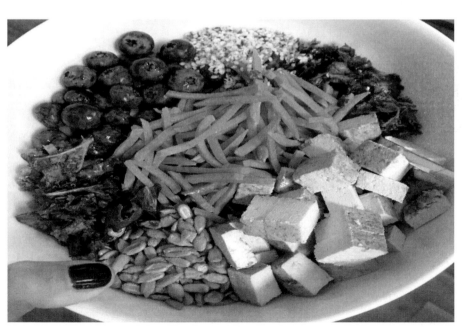

4.1 The Best Foods to Eat While Intermittent Fasting

Water

If we're going hungry for an extended period, hydration becomes even more important. When we fast, the sugar stored in our liver becomes our body's preferred energy source (glycogen). We lose a large amount of fluid and electrolytes as we burn this energy. As a result, it's important to consume at least 8 cups of water a day. Not only can this avoid dehydration, but it will also improve blood circulation, muscle and joint support, and cognitive function.

Minimally-processed grains

Carbs, whether you like them or not, are a necessary part of life. It's also important to consider how to eat enough calories without being excessively satiated while fasting strategically. Choose foods that are easy to digest, such as whole-grain bread and crackers. These will also provide an excellent source of energy when on the go.

Coffee

If you've been putting off starting this diet since you can't live without coffee, there's good news: you can. Coffee is a calorie-free beverage in its natural state, so you can drink it even if you're fasting. Simply leave out the syrups, creamers, and other flavors.

Lentils

Half a cup of lentils provides almost a third of your regular fiber requirements. They're also high in iron (approximately 15% of your daily requirement), so women can eat plenty of them.

Strawberries

Looking for a tasty way to increase your fiber intake? Go for the raspberries. These berries have eight grams of fiber per cup, which lets you consume more whole fruits.

Hummus

For those who are intermittently fasting, this smooth, tasty dip is a perfect plant-based protein source. It also works well as a mayonnaise replacement. Hummus is a perfect mini-meal to have during the middle of your 8-hour eating window when you're doing the 16:8 intermittent fast.

Potatoes

White potatoes, like our minimally processed grains, are relatively easy to digest. You should combine them with only a protein source for something like a post-workout snack to recharge your muscles if you're working out and intermittently fasting. Another advantage of having potatoes in your IF diet is that they form a complex carbohydrate that feeds your gut bacteria when they cool.

Wild-caught salmon

With a shorter meal window, it's more important than ever to make sure you're getting your minerals and vitamins from every bite. It's rich in the omega-3 fatty acids EPA and DHA, which are good for the brain. Serve it with your favorite vegetables (the best is coconut oil) for a fast (and delicious) super food dinner.

Milk with added vitamin D

Adults require approximately 1,000 milligrams of calcium a day, which is about 3 glasses of milk. Although most people do not drink three glasses of milk a day, high-calcium foods should also be prioritized. It's great in smoothies and cereal. If you are lactose intolerant, go for tofu or leafy greens such as kale instead.

Nuts

They are beneficial to your health. Nut intake was linked to a lower risk of heart disease, Type 2 diabetes, and overall mortality in a prospective trial published in the British Journal of Nutrition. So, pack some in your purse and keep them around when you're within your feeding window.

4.2 Types of Intermittent Fasting

Diets are becoming increasingly common as a means of losing weight, avoiding illness, and increasing longevity. However, based on your lifestyle and priorities, there are many choices.

Which intermittent fasting type is right for you?

"Tell me what to eat," a registered dietitian sometimes hears. "Tell me when not to eat," they may be hearing now. It's called intermittent fasting (IF), and it's a dietary strategy that includes interspersing scheduled fasting times with daily meals. This diet, according to proponents, is the secret to long-term weight loss, improved metabolic health, and a long lifespan.

4.3 The Proposed Health Benefits of Intermittent Fasting

When it comes to losing weight, there are two theories as to why IF might be successful. The first is that "fasting cycles create a net calorie deficit, and as a result, you lose weight," says Rekha Kumar, MD, an endocrinologist, diabetes, and metabolism specialist at Weill Cornell Medicine and New York-Presbyterian in New York City. The other definition is more difficult to grasp: She assumes that the so-called "plateau phenomenon" can be avoided by following this approach.

You may recall the popular "Biggest Loser" report published in the journal Obesity in August 2016. After six years, the researchers found that, after the initial remarkable weight loss, the participants had recovered the majority of their weight and that their metabolic rates had slowed, resulting in them burning much fewer calories than would be expected.

While more research on the efficacy and safety of IF is required, one of its touted benefits is that it may prevent metabolic sputtering. "Most people who want to lose weight by diet and exercise end up falling off the wagon and gaining weight. Hormones that encourage weight gain, such as appetite hormones, are activated, and it's thought that intermittent fasting (IF) will help avoid this metabolic adaptation," says Dr. Kumar. Normal eating patterns in IF "trick" the body into weight loss until it reaches a plateau.

So, does it help you lose weight? Proponents of the proposal have agreed with a simple yes based on anecdotal proof. "For people who can stick to IF, it works," Kumar says. However, proponents of the method argue that it is about much more than just getting a lean body. Lori Shemek, Ph.D., a Dallas diet and weight loss specialist and author of How to Combat FATflammation, tells clients that IF can increase insulin sensitivity (lowering the risk of type 2 diabetes), minimize inflammation, and "boost longevity by improving the health of your mitochondria" according to her.

Obese adults who followed IF for eight weeks lost an average of 12 pounds while also lowering their total cholesterol, "bad" LDL cholesterol, and systolic blood pressure.

The journal Nutrition and Healthy Aging published a study in June 2018 that showed that 12 weeks of IF did not impact cholesterol levels, but it did help with weight loss and lower systolic blood pressure. In October 2019, the journal Nutrients published a study of 11 IF trials in overweight and obese adults that lasted at least eight weeks. Nine of those researchers found that an IF program was just as successful in helping people lose weight and fat as conventional dieting instead of limiting calories every day.

However, it's worth noting that researching human longevity is far more complicated than studying weight loss. That's why, as in a report published in June 2018 in the journal Current Biology, much of the research that indicates IF facilitates a longer life span has indeed been done in animals, including fruit flies. Another study published in the New England Journal of Medicine in December 2019 indicated that the metabolic benefit of Intermittent Fasting is that it brings your body into a state of ketosis (the keto diet's metabolic state), where fat is burned instead of carbohydrates for energy. According to the researchers, the idea that ketones can activate the body's repair system, eventually protecting against illness and aging, goes further than weight loss effects.

It's also vital to hold the expectations in check. Since a lot of research is done on animals, it's more difficult to apply the findings to humans, who are more free-thinking and then have to deal with the consequences of lifestyle problems like work stress, crazy routines, emotional eating, and hunger pangs, to name a few — that can make it difficult to stick to a diet. IF might be promising, but it's "actually no more successful than any other diet," according to a 2018 research.

4.4 Who Shouldn't Try Intermittent Fasting

Not everyone can (or wants to) participate in IF. Women who are pregnant or attempting to be pregnant (extended fasting cycles can throw off the menstrual cycle), diabetics (blood sugar may drop too low in the absence of food), and anyone taking several drugs (food, or lack thereof, can affect dosage and absorption), according to Kumar. Also, if you've got a background in eating disorders, adding times where you're "not allowed" to eat might set you up for a dangerous relapse.

It's important to be aware that IF has any side effects. Since low blood sugar can mess with your mood, you can be cranky — "hanger" is true — during fasting times. When you do eat, you must try to eat a healthy diet. "One idea is that if you fasted for two days, it would be hard to make up a calorie deficit, but in our culture, with access to calorie-dense foods, you could do it," Kumar says. Concentrate on nutrient-dense foods such as lean meats, vegetables, whole grains, legumes, and fruits. Expect low energy, bloating, and hunger pangs for the first few weeks as the body changes, says Shemek.

4.5 Types of Intermittent Fasting

There are a lot of ways to perform IF, which is fantastic. If this is something you're interested in, you can choose the kind that best suits your needs, increasing your chances of success. Here are seven of them:

1. Fasting

This is among the most widely used IF techniques. The plan is to normally eat for five days (without counting calories) and then consume 500 or 600 calories per day for men and women, respectively, for the remaining two days. The fasting days can be any days you like.

Short fasting periods are thought to keep you compliant; if you get hungry on a fast day, just think of tomorrow when you can "feast" again. "Some people think, 'I can do something for two days, but cutting back on what I eat for seven days is too much,' Kumar says. For these individuals, a 5:2 solution might be preferable to calorie restriction during the week.

However, the writers of The FastDiet warn against fasting on days when you're doing a bunch of intense exercises. If you're training for cycling or running a race (or a high-mileage week), consult a sports nutritionist to see if this style of fasting will fit with your training schedule.

2. Time-Restricted Fasting

This form of IF requires you to pick an eating window each day, which should leave you with a 14 to 16 hour fast. (Shemek advises women to fast for no more than 14 hours a day due to hormonal concerns.) "Fasting encourages autophagy, the body's normal 'cellular housekeeping' mechanism that starts when liver glycogen is exhausted and clears debris and other items that get in the way of mitochondrial health," Shemek says. According to her, doing so can help maximize fat cell metabolism and optimize insulin function.

Set your eating window, for example, from 9 a.m. to 5 p.m. to make this work. According to Kumar, this works particularly well for someone who has a family who enjoys an early dinner anyway. Then there's the fact that most of the time spent fasting is spent sleeping. (Depending on when you scheduled your window, you also don't have to "skip" any meals.) However, this is contingent on your ability to be consistent. Regular fasting cycles might not be for you if your schedule is constantly changing or if you want or need the freedom to go out to brunch on occasion, go on a dinner date, or go to happy hour.

3. Overnight Fasting

This method is the most basic of the lot, and it entails fasting for 12 hours every day. Consider the following scenario: Choose to avoid eating by 7 p.m. after dinner and start eating at 7 a.m.

the next morning with breakfast. At the 12-hour mark, autophagy still occurs, but the cellular benefits are milder, according to Shemek. This is the bare minimum of fasting periods she advises.

This approach has the advantage of being simple to implement. You still don't have to miss meals; what you're doing is cutting out a bedtime snack. However, this approach does not completely harness the benefits of fasting. If you're fasting to lose weight, a smaller fasting window ensures you'll have more time to eat, which does not help you consume fewer calories.

4. Eat Stop Eat

Brad Pilon's strategy differs from others in that it emphasizes versatility. Simply put, he emphasizes that fasting is simply abstaining from food for some time. You agree to a resistance training regimen and one or two 24-hour fasts per week. "When the fast is done, I want you to eat responsibly and live as though it never happened. That is everything there is to it.

Eating wisely entails returning to a regular eating routine in which you don't binge because you've fasted, but you still don't starve yourself or consume less than you require. Fat loss is best achieved by combining intermittent fasting with routine weight training, according to Pilon. You will consume a significantly higher number of calories on the remaining five or six non-fasting days if you go on one or two 24-hour fasts throughout the week. He claims that this makes it simpler and more fun to finish the week with a calorific deficit without being compelled to go on a strict diet.

5. Whole-Day Fasting

You only eat once a day here. According to Shemek, some people prefer to eat dinners and then not consume food again till the next day's dinner. That means you'll be fasting for 24 hours. This is not the same as the 5:2 form. Fasting times are usually 24 hours (lunch to lunch or dinner to dinner), while 5:2 requires a 36-hour fast. (For example, you could eat dinner on Sunday, then go on a 500-600 calorie fast on Monday before breaking it with breakfast on Tuesday.)

The benefit is that, if exercised for weight loss, eating an entire day's worth of calories in one sitting is extremely difficult (though not impossible). The downside of this strategy is that it's difficult to get all of the body's nutrients with only one meal. Not to mention, sticking to this strategy is difficult. By the time dinner arrives, you may be ravenous, leading you to consume less-than-healthy, calorie-dense foods. Consider this: When you're hungry, broccoli isn't exactly the first thing that comes to mind. According to Shemek, many people drink too much coffee to satisfy their appetite, disrupting their sleep. If you don't eat, you can experience brain fog during the day.

6. Alternate-Day Fasting

Krista Varady popularized this method. People can fast every other day fast, comprising 25% of their daily calorie requirements (approximately 500 calories) and non-fasting days being regular eating days. This is a common weight-loss strategy. In reality, Dr. Varady and the team found that alternate-day fasting successfully helped obese adults lose weight in a limited study published in Nutrition Journal. By week two, the participants' side effects (such as hunger) had subsided, and by week four, they felt more relaxed on a diet.

The downside is that participants said they were never really "complete" during the 8 weeks of the study, making sticking to this plan difficult.

7. Choose-Your-Day Fasting

It's more like a pick-your-own adventure here. According to Shemek, you can do time-restricted fasting every other day or once or twice a week. That means you could have a regular day of eating on Sunday, stop eating by 8 p.m., and start eating again at noon on Monday. It's the equivalent of missing breakfast a few times a week.

Chapter 5: Darkside of intermittent fasting

As previously stated, the benefits of intermittent fasting are being studied, but there are some positive results. However, there is more than enough anecdotal evidence that intermittent fasting has some potentially harmful side effects, and you must discuss them with your doctor before embarking on an intermittent fasting eating plan.

Here are ten red flags to be aware of. If you experience any other side effects, you should immediately pause intermittent fasting and consult with your doctor or even a nutritionist before continuing.

5.1 Are you are hungry?

We're not sure if "hungriness" is a real term, but it is undoubtedly a real sensation. This is the grumpiness, irritability, or general irritability from not eating while your body indicates that you are hungry. Training the body to go Sixteen hours without food requires some practice, and some people's bodies can never be satisfied with eating within such a narrow window. In principle, you shouldn't be hungry first thing every morning if you eat enough protein later during the day or night. If you are, that's a sign that you need to undergo some dietary changes during your calorie intake cycle to stop being a total jerk—or that's a sign that fasting isn't working for you. Not eating for long periods might not be suitable for certain people (e.g., those who work out a lot), worth considering. Don't try to push it.

You can feel increased hunger if you minimize your calorie consumption or go long stretches without eating. Some 112 people were randomly allocated to either an intermittent energy limitation category in a survey. For a year, they ate 400 and perhaps 600 calories on two non-consecutive days per week. These individuals reported feeling hungrier than those who followed a low-calorie diet with constant calorie restriction. According to studies, hunger is a common symptom people encounter within the first few days of such a fasting regimen.

In a 2020 survey, 1,422 people took part in fasting regimens that lasted 4–21 days. Only in the first several days of the regimens did they experience hunger symptoms. As a result, hunger symptoms can fade as your body adjusts to normal fasting periods.

5.2 Fatigue or fogging of the mind

Have you ever woken up in the middle of the morning, yawning uncontrollably, only to realize you'd forgotten to eat breakfast? Most people do intermittent fasting by skipping breakfast; noticing that you're always tired or making mistakes because of brain fog signifies that you're not consuming the right foods throughout non-fasting hours. Fasting isn't working for you. You should pay more attention to what you're putting into your body. You can eat whatever you want on intermittent fasting, but you really should still fuel it with nutritious foods that make you feel safe and strong. Listen to your body if you feel *much* healthier eating breakfast most days.

Intermittent fasting can make you feel exhausted and weak due to low blood sugar. In addition, intermittent fasting can cause sleep disturbances in some people, resulting in fatigue during the day. On the other hand, some studies have shown intermittent fasting to reduce fatigue, particularly as your body adapts to daily fasting periods.

5.3 Obsessions with food

Being on a restricted diet may affect your relationship with food. While some people enjoy the strictness of intermittent fasting, others can find themselves obsessing about what they should eat and how many calories should consume. Spending too much time worrying about the quality and quantity of the food daily can lead to orthorexia, an eating disorder. As per the National Eating Disorders Association, orthorexia is a condition where you place such a high value on "right" or "healthy" eating to hurt your overall health. The aim of any diet should be to form a safe, meaningful relationship with food, not to lose weight.

5.4 A low blood sugar level

Suppose you experience constant nausea, headache, or dizziness while on the intermittent fasting diet; it's a red flag that your blood sugar is out of whack. People with diabetes may avoid any form of a fasting diet for this purpose, as previously stated by WH: Hypoglycemia, a risky condition for those with insulin and otherwise thyroid issues, may be caused by intermittent fasting.

5.5 Hair Loss

Is this for real? Yes. Hair loss can be caused by unexpected weight loss or even an absence of appropriate nutrients, particularly protein and B vitamins. Although intermittent fasting (IF) does not always result in nutritional loss, it is more difficult to eat a well-balanced diet when you are cramming a full day's worth of eating into a few hours. Re-evaluate the nutrient quality of the daily meals and consult with the doctor about whether this is a good decision if you notice more hair falling out from the shower than normal.

5.6 Constipation

Is it all backed up? It's possible that intermittent fasting is to blame. "If you don't get enough fluid, vitamins, proteins, or fiber, any deficiency can reduce an upset stomach. So, if you've begun an intermittent fasting diet and aren't having normal bowel movements, it's time to put your plan on hold and talk to a nutritionist or doctor about what's going on.

5.7 Unhealthy eating habits

Even if IF (intermittent fasting) does not cause a severe illness such as orthorexia, it may also lead to poor eating behaviors. You also can find yourself making poor nutritional decisions during non-fasting hours, in addition to not having enough nutrients. "The biggest concern is that you'll start binge-eating because you're so hungry," Charlie Seltzer. If this describes you, you may benefit from working with such an RD to develop a plan that doesn't require you to limit your eating hours instead and focuses on providing your body with the nutrients it needs every day, not just at those hours.

5.8 Sleep deprivation

According to some studies, sleep disturbances, including an inability to fall or remain asleep, are among the common side effects of intermittent fasting. In a 2020 survey, 1,422 people took part in fasting regimens that lasted 4–21 days. Fasting caused sleep disturbances in 15% of the participants, according to the report. This was mentioned more often than other side effects. Since your body excretes large quantities of water and salt through the urine, fatigue can be more normal in the early days of even an intermittent fasting regimen. Dehydration, as well as low salt levels, can result as a result of this.

Other studies, on the other hand, have found that intermittent fasting has little effect on sleep. Research published in 2021 looked at 31 obese people who fasted on alternating days while still eating a low-carb diet over six months. According to the report, this routine did not affect sleep quality and duration or insomnia severity. Similar findings were found in a study conducted in 2021.

Many people report better sleep patterns when doing IF, probably because IF allows curbing late-night snacking behaviors, leading to an inability to drift off to sleep because the stomach is still digesting the 10 p.m. snack. However, some evidence suggests that the opposite is true. Evidence suggests that circadian rhythms intermittent fasting (daytime fasting) reduces rapid-eye-movement (REM) sleep, according to a study published in the journal Science and Nature of Sleep in 2018. According to the Harvard Business Review, getting sufficient REM sleep has been related to various health effects, including improved memory, cognition, and attention. It's unclear why this is the case.

If you're having trouble falling or staying asleep after starting an IF (intermittent fasting) balanced diet, pause and consult a professional to ensure you're not harming your health.

5.9   Constant Changes in Mood

It'd be odd if you didn't have mood swings or hungriness throughout intermittent fasting, at least at first. Although some people experience a significant increase in energy or motivation after adjusting to fasting, it's important to keep in mind that it's still a restricted diet. Feeling obliged to stick to it might make you depressed, particularly if you're isolating yourself from friends or family due to your dietary restrictions. Stop and speak with a licensed dietitian, counselor, or wellness coach right away if you're feeling down, nervous, or discouraged about intermittent fasting. They might assist you in developing a fasting regimen that is more suitable for your body and mind.

When people practice intermittent fasting, they can experience irritability as well as other mood swings. When the blood sugar levels are poor, you can become irritable. Hypoglycemia, or low blood sugar, can occur throughout periods with calorie restriction or fasting. Irritability, anxiety, and low focus are all possible outcomes. A 2016 study of 52 women was found during an eighteen-hour fasting cycle, and participants were substantially more irritable than after a non-fasting period. Interestingly, the researchers discovered that, while the women were irritable at the end of the fasting era, they also felt a greater sense of accomplishment, dignity, and self-control than they did initially.

5.10 Lightheadedness and headaches

Intermittent fasting is also linked with headaches. They usually happen in those last few days or even a fasting regimen. In a study published in 2020, researchers looked through 18 studies involving people who practiced intermittent fasting. Any participants in the four studies who reported side effects said they had moderate headaches.

Researchers also discovered that "fasting headaches" are normally located throughout the brain's frontal area, with mild to moderate pain in severity.

Furthermore, people who suffer from headaches are often more likely to suffer from headaches when fasting than those that do not. According to research, low blood sugar and caffeine withdrawal can lead to headaches throughout intermittent fasting.

5.11 Problems with digestion

If you are doing intermittent fasting, you can experience digestive problems such as constipation, diarrhea, nausea, and bloating. The reduction of food intake that certain intermittent fasting regimens entail can have a detrimental impact on your digestion, resulting in constipation and other unpleasant side effects. Additionally, dietary changes associated with intermittent fasting programs can result in bloating and diarrhea. Constipation may be exacerbated by dehydration, another popular side effect of intermittent fasting. As a result, it is important to remain well hydrated while fasting intermittently. Constipation can be avoided by eating nutrient-dense, fiber-rich foods.

5.12 Bad Brea

Bad breath is also an unwanted side effect that some people experience when they fast intermittently. Lack salivary flow and an increase in acetone throughout the breath trigger this. Fasting allows the body to burn fat as a source of energy. Since acetone would be a by-product of fat metabolism, it rises in the blood and breath when you fast.

Dehydration, a sign of intermittent fasting, may also trigger a dry mouth, leading to bad breath.

5.13 Dehydration

As previously mentioned, the body releases a lot of water and salt in the urine during the first few days of fasting. Natural diuresis, also known as fasting natriuresis, is the name given to this operation. You might become dehydrated if something happens with you and you do not restore the fluids and electrolytes lost by urine. In addition, people who practice intermittent fasting can fail to drink or drink insufficiently. This is particularly true when you first start an intermittent fasting program. Drink water during the day and keep an eye on the color of your urine to stay properly hydrated. It should ideally be the color of pale lemonade. You could be dehydrated if your urine is dark in color.

5.14 Malnutrition

Intermittent fasting, if performed incorrectly, will result in malnutrition. Malnutrition can occur when an individual fast for long periods and does not replenish the body with enough nutrients. The same can be said for unplanned, long-term energy restriction diets. On different forms of intermittent fasting systems, people can usually fulfill their calorie and nutrient requirements. However, suppose you do not properly schedule or execute the fasting regimen for a long time or intentionally limit calories to an excessive amount. In that case, you risk malnutrition and other health problems. That is why, when fasting intermittently, it is important to eat a well-balanced, healthy diet. Make sure you are not restricting your calorie consumption too much.

A healthcare professional familiar with intermittent fasting will assist you in developing a health plan that offers the right number of calories and nutrients for you.

Chapter 6: Tips and Tricks for Intermittent Fasting

6.1. Tips to follow while Intermittent Fasting

1. Eat Well During the Eating Window

It has been said that everyone can fast, but still, it takes intelligence to crack it. After breaking a fast, what an individual eats is extremely important. A large green salad bowl with raw vegetables dipped in olive oil and steamed broccoli, spinach, or baked yam will be the ideal breakfast meal. Vegetables are commonly favored because they are low in calories and high in nutrients. Often, aim to consume a nutritious diet with a variety of nutrients during the eating window.

2. Add Fiber to Your Diet

Women over 50 may find intermittent fasting difficult, particularly if they have not encountered hunger for several hours per day. During the eating window, eating foods high in fiber and protein may help combat this issue. Fiber makes you feel complete and will help you avoid a blood sugar drop. Pasta, whole-grain bread, nuts, as well as beans are also good sources of fiber.

3. Crescendo Fasting is good for a start.

Beginner fasters should begin with the crescendo approach because it establishes more manageable objectives. It is the preferred method of fasting for women because it ensures that hormone levels do not fluctuate excessively. This technique ensures beginners get the most from intermittent fasting because it is a much gentler way to intermittent fasting.

4. Check the hormone levels regularly.

Intermittent fasting in various forms appears to be healthy for women. However, serious side effects like increased appetite, mood swings, decreased concentration, and bad breath has been documented in some studies. Whether some women have confirmed a complete cessation of their menstrual cycle. As a result, it's critical that women who are experiencing a quick monitor their hormones regularly. If a woman's mood or health condition changes significantly, she should stop fasting immediately and see a doctor.

5. Decide how you'd like to fast.

Intermittent fasting, as previously stated, is a cyclical cycle of fasting that includes calorie restriction or food abstinence, accompanied by food intake. We have various intermittent fasting plans based on this definition. Longer periods of fasting, on the other hand, may result in the development of gallstones. Women, irrespective of their weight, are at a higher risk. It's also possible that skipping breakfast isn't the best option for everybody. According to a report published by the European

Society of Cardiology, such habit may be linked to atherosclerosis, a disease marked by artery narrowing and hardening.

If you want to miss breakfast, make sure to stay hydrated during the day and start slowly, paying attention to body language for energy crashes. If you're having trouble getting to your next meal and finding it difficult to work in the morning with no food, you might want to reconsider your fasting strategy.

6. Maintain as much of a routine as possible

Your favorite fasting method is just as important as your dedication to the schedule. You want to pick an intermittent fasting regimen that you can stick to as much as possible.

These pointers can be useful:

Make dinner the last meal so that your fasting time is extended.

Make a schedule for the week's events. Switch your fasting time the day before if you intend to join a birthday lunch on Friday.

Keep yourself occupied so that you don't end up grabbing nutrition throughout the middle of your fast.

Do you want to exercise? If possible, do after the quick.

7. Maintain hydration

Hunger is one of the immediate consequences of intermittent fasting because you're more likely to jeopardize your

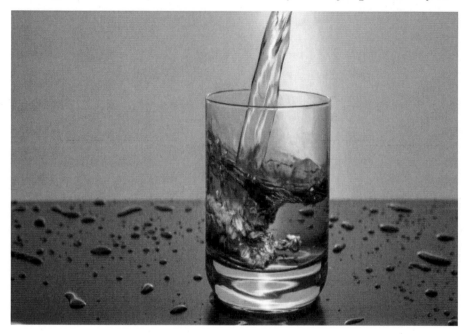

performance when you're hungry. Drink anything in between to stop it IF it allows you to drink herbal teas, tea, and water while fasting. You can also try a drink with alkalizing greens like wheatgrass, kale, broccoli, spirulina, butternut squash, collard greens, green beans, beet greens, and celery can help you refuel. You will have more energy and improved cognitive performance, better digestion, and less inflammation if you keep your body slightly alkaline.

8. Maintain Portion Control.

You don't have the luxury of obesity during your non-fast time because you're on an intermittent fasting diet. This merely negates the advantages of intermittent fasting.

Portion control is still essential, but it can be difficult when your stomach is grumbling. One strategy is to space out your meals, so you don't have to consume big portions during your non-fast period.

Consider the following plan if you have an 8-hour feeding window:

- Eat the first regular meal within the first hour.

- During the second hour, eat a small snack.

- Eat your second regular meal at the third hour.

- Get another quick snack at the fifth hour.

- Eat the last usual meal at the seventh hour.

- Between these meals, drink plenty of water and, if it works, have used a smaller plate with improved portion control.

9. Consume the Correct Foods

Eating the right foods goes hand in hand with portion control. When IF leaves you hungry, you can reach for microwaveable meals or the nearest burger-and-fry joint. You can also drink sweetened drinks for the flavor or because you feel you need to raise your carbohydrate intake. Both of these will not provide you with the desired intermittent fasting performance. Processed foods, especially those that are ultra-processed, can make you feel even hungrier. Worse, you're growing the chances of developing metabolic problems, such as obesity.

Here are some healthy food suggestions:

Avocados and salmon are good sources of healthy fats.

Grass-fed beef, nutritious tofu, grains, peas, and lentils are good sources of nutritious, lean protein.

Pile leafy greens on your plate.

As a snack, eat some nuts.

Consider making nutritious food substitutions.

In between fasting times, some people choose to eat a low-carb, low-calorie plan to maintain fat burning and reduce the risk of weight gain. One example is the ketogenic diet.

10. Sleep Well

Sleep deprivation can also cause you to lose or not achieve your desirable intermittent fasting performance. Sleep deprivation can cause various issues, including a loss of control over calorie consumption and weight. It can increase the development of ghrelin, a hormone that increases appetite. It can also reduce the release of leptin, a hormone that helps to control hunger.

Sleep deprivation can cause you to crave more cookies or other sweets. This is because it may stimulate endocannabinoid, the same form of lipid that marijuana stimulates. A minimum of eight hours of sleep is an optimal goal to strive for. If you're having trouble sleeping, make sure you're practicing healthy sleep habits like not using devices (blue light) until bed and not drinking caffeine until 4–6 hours of going to bed.

6.2   Weight Loss tips

The following suggestions will assist you in losing weight more quickly.

1. Obtain Enough Rest

The appetite hormones leptin and ghrelin are strongly influenced by sleep. So make sure you get 6-8 hours of sleep every day to keep your appetite in check and stop overeating.

2. Strengthen the body.

Intermittent fasting combined with strength and weight training can speed up weight loss and improve muscle mass.

3. Sugar consumption should be reduced.

Sugars and carbohydrates play a significant role in weight gain and can reduce the benefits of intermittent fasting. As a result, sugary foods and beverages should be avoided.

4. Keep a food diary

Keeping a food log will assist you in keeping track of your calories, including weight loss while dieting. This will assist you in regulating your eating habits and daily schedule following your needs, allowing you to optimize your gains.

5. Take a probiotic supplement.

Probiotics are known to help with digestive health, gut microbiome restoration, and immune system support. So, to stay balanced during intermittent fasting, be sure to bring probiotic supplements. Women of all ages may benefit from intermittent fasting. If you are a woman over 50 who wants to lose the last few stubborn pounds, try intermittent fasting.

Chapter 7: Psychological effects of intermittent fasting

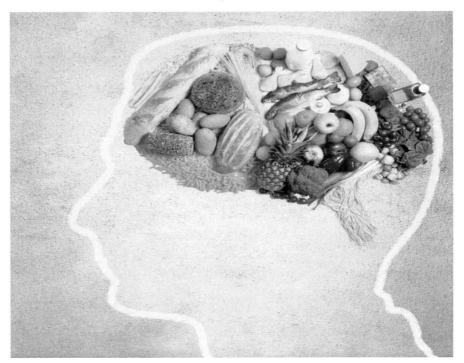

7.1 It has the potential to affect your mood.

If you've been too hungry, and who hasn't? You're well aware that an empty stomach can lead to irritability and rage. Spend enough time without food, thanks to intermittent fasting, and your mood will begin to change. Are you irritable? This is due to low blood sugar levels and "a spike in cortisol (the stress hormone)," which occurs when people become overly hungry. Your blood sugar falls eventually spikes when "feasting" can be particularly dangerous for people with diabetes because they can lead to a loss of blood glucose regulation and interfere with diabetes treatment and insulin requirements. (It is worth noting that low-carb diets such as the keto diet can benefit people with diabetes). Are you combative? That also appears to be right. "There seems to be a hormone named neuropeptide Y which causes people to be more aggressive when they're really hungry," Albers-Bowling says, "going back to caveman days when you just got to eat if you had been fighting or your dinner."

7.2   It may make you feel even more anxious.

The higher the level of cortisol in your body, the further likely you are to be depressed. According to some research, "there is some evidence that restricting dietary activity increases a stress hormone cortisol, which can induce changes in food preferences, cravings, and mood." High cortisol levels also have been related to increased fat accumulation, so IF can work against you if you're looking to lose weight.

7.3   It can make you tired

Although a small pilot study showed which intermittent fasting could boost your night, other research suggests that it is much more likely to cause sleep problems. As per a study in the journal Science and Nature of Sleep, fasting will reduce REM sleep (the super intense healing shut-eye), leading to the body's increase in cortisol and insulin. (The good news is that you can eat your path to improve sleep). Depending on the intermittent fasting strategy you use, you can avoid eating several hours before bedtime, which is a good thing because eating right before bedtime is bad for your health, leading to weight gain, acid reflux, excessive gas, and sleeping problems. However, an empty, growling stomach will make sleeping difficult.

And, let's face it, adequate sleep is important for overall mental health: "Changes in sleep behavior, quality, and length can lead to fatigue but mostly affect your mood the next day," says a researcher. (On that note, this is how your brain feels when you do not get enough sleep).

7.4   It can make you lonely

When you're unable to feed for extended periods, it can impact food-related social situations between friends and family. According to the American Psychological Association, losing out again on friend time may lead to feelings of loneliness and social alienation, leading to depression. As per the National Eating Disorders Association, those with anorexia report having fewer mates, social interests, and social support because of their diet restrictions.

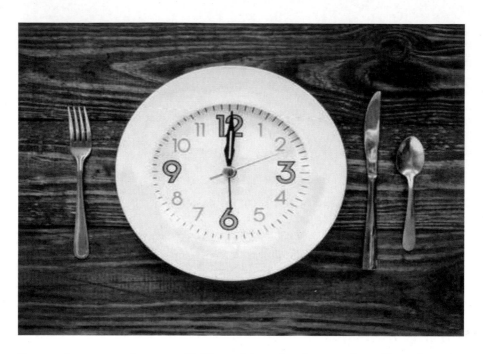

It can increase the possibility of developing eating disorders in some people. Intermittent fasting's rigid rules about once you can and can't eat, according to the researchers, may be upsetting for someone who has had or is at risk of having an eating disorder. "At the most fundamental level, anorexia is about imposing dietary restrictions and restrictive guidelines, ignoring hunger yet fullness, and obsessing over food, all of whom can be perpetuated and compounded by Intermittent Fasting." (Also, have you ever studied orthorexia? It is an eating disorder masquerading as a balanced eating plan.) According to the researcher, the diet can also lead to "fear of losing control (with food)" or "overeating on non-restricted days." Binge eating disorder manifests itself in both of these ways. In reality, one study showed that women who reduced the caloric intake by 70% for four days but instead ate "normally" over three days had more eating-related feelings, a greater fear of losing control, and a more regular tendency for overeating throughout non-restricted hunger for just a total of four weeks. According to Albers-Bowling, Intermittent Fasting may also mask a current eating disorder. "When you say, 'Oh, I'm avoiding eating because I'm on the new fasting dieting,' people don't seem concerned. "

If you cannot take your mind off the diet or find yourself eating more than you'd if you've not fasted, intermittent fasting probably isn't for you. According to experts, intermittent fasting should be avoided entirely if you have a history of disordered eating or a poor relationship to food.

According to Hertz, intermittent fasting could be detrimental to anyone's relationship to food, but it is particularly dangerous for those with a history of disordered eating. "This is because they have a higher chance of abusing the rules and regulations to allow and exacerbate their eating disorder."

7.5   It can have an impact on your cognitive abilities

According to a study, fasting over long periods will cause you to make further rash, short-term decisions. You adjust the neurotransmitters, which are accessible throughout the brain when you fast. "As a result, restricting foods which increase serotonin levels can result in less of a feel-good chemical in your brain," which can make you more impulsive. Consider this when making food choices. In the meantime, another study of mice reported in the Published In the journal of Scientific Studies in Biosciences indicates that intermittent fasting may increase levels from certain neurotransmitters, such as serotonin, and improve learning and memory. There's contradictory evidence of the latest studies on intermittent fasting and arguments made in this paper. If you have a headache? The same. Unfortunately, there is still a ton about intermittent fasting that we do not fully comprehend.

7.6   Your perception of hunger might change

Intermittent fasting is, at its heart, about gaining mental power over hunger and, in so doing, ignoring the body's hunger signals (which, by the way, are generate by a hormone named ghrelin). According to new studies, intermittent fasting can aid with weight loss by lowering appetite and decreasing your hunger hormone ghrelin. According to animal studies, these (intermittent fasting) IF-induced increases in ghrelin can also increase dopamine levels (pleasure hormone) in the brain.

Hunger, on the other hand, is like a noisy knock on your front gate. "When you want to avoid the queues, it's as if you're covering your ears while saying, "I don't hear you; if only I wait long enough, they'll go away. Hunger appears to pound harder in the hopes of eliciting a response. If you ignore hunger signals, they will eventually stop knocking. This has a long-term negative impact on your relationship with hunger.

Chapter No. 8 Meal plan and Recipes

If you're new to fasting, starting only by eating between 8 a.m. and 6 p.m. is a wonderful way to get your feet wet.

8.1 Meal Plan

The plan involves eating all of your meals and some snacks while still fasting for 14 hours in 24 hours.

To stop a blood-sugar roller coaster, opt for a green smoothie rather than a high-carb fruit smoothie in the morning. To fill you up until lunch, include plenty of healthy fats.

Ingredients:

- Avocado 1

- Coconut milk 1 cup

- Blueberries 1 small handful

- Spinach, chard, or kale 1 cup

- Chia seeds 1 tbsp

Instructions

1. Blend all of the ingredients in a blender and enjoy

AT 12 P.M., GRASS-FED BURGERS

Grass-fed liver burgers are among the favorite weekday lunch options, and they're super easy to prepare ahead of time to enjoy throughout the week. This can be served over a bed of dark leafy greens with an easy homemade dressing for a B vitamin-rich meal that promotes healthy methylation and detox paths.

Ingredients:

- Ground grass-fed beef liver ½ lb.

- Ground grass-fed beef ½ lb.

- Garlic powder½ tsp

- Cumin powder ½ tsp

- Sea salt and pepper as taste

- Desired cooking oil

Instructions

1. In a mixing bowl, combine all ingredients and shape them into desired size patties.

2. Heat the cooking oil in a skillet over medium-high heat.

3. Cook burgers in a skillet until cooked to your taste.

4. Refrigerate in an airtight jar and use for four days.

SNACK: FAT BOMBS CINNAMON ROLL AT 2:30 P.M.

Fat bombs will satisfy your sweet tooth while supplying sufficient healthy fats to keep you going until dinner, and they taste just like cinnamon rolls.

INGREDIENTS:

- Coconut cream ½ cup

- Cinnamon 1 tsp

- Coconut oil 1 tbsp

- Almond butter 2 tbsp

Instructions

1. Mix half tsp cinnamon and coconut cream

2. Line parchment paper and an 8-by-8 square inch pan and spread cinnamon mixture and coconut cream at the bottom

3. Blend half tsp of cinnamon, almond butter, and coconut oil and spread it over the layer mentioned above.

4. Cut into bars or squares as you like but after freezing for ten minutes.

DINNER: VEGGIES AND SALMON AT 5:30 P.M.

Salmon is an outstanding source of healthy omega-3 fats, and the antioxidants are high in dark green veggies, such as kale and broccoli. Salmon is one of my personal favorites for its taste and nutrient density, but you can pick any wild seafood of your choice. Serve your favorite greens in coconut oil together and have a simple superfood meal. Serve them fast and easy.

INGREDIENTS:

- Salmon or any other fish of choice 1 lb.

- Fresh lemon juice 2 tbsp

- Ghee 2 tbsp

- Clove's garlic, thinly diced 4

Instructions

1. Preheat the oven to 400 degrees Fahrenheit.

2. Combine the lemon juice, garlic, and ghee in a mixing bowl.

3. Wrap the salmon in foil and drizzle the ghee and lemon mixture over it.

4. Put the salmon over a baking sheet and wrap it in foil.

5. Bake for 15 minutes or until the salmon is finished.

6. You can roast vegetables alongside the salmon on a separate baking sheet if your oven requires it.

2. INTERMEDIATE FASTING MEAL PLAN.

This plan allows you to only eat for full 18-hour fasting within 24 hours between 12 p.m. and 6 p.m.

Even if you skip breakfast, staying hydrated is still important. Always drink plenty of water. You can also use herbal tea (most of the specialists agree that coffee does not break quickly.) It has been shown that the catechins in tea enhance the effects of fasting by reducing Ghrelin's hunger hormone further until lunch, and you don't feel deprived.

You must make sure that your first meal is healthy enough because you have extended your fasting period for another four hours. The burger of the 8-to-6 plan works fine, and with your dressage or top of an avocado, you can add more fats.

Seeds and nuts make good, high-fat snacks that can be eaten at approximately 2:30. Before taking them, natural enzymes like phytates that can contribute to digestive problems can be neutralized. Eat dinner at 5:30 p.m. as well as eight to six windows; it's a great option to have dinner in some kind of wild fish or other smooth protein springs with vegetables.

- First meal: Grass-fed burger with avocado at midnight.

- Snack: seeds and nuts, at 2:30 p.m.

- Second meal: veggies and Salmon, at 5:30 p.m.

3. ADVANCED: THE REVISED 2-DAY MEAL PLAN.

Eat clean for any five days a week for this plan. Two days later, limit your calories to a maximum of 700 every day. Calorie restriction offers many of the same advantages for a whole day as fasting.

You will have to make sure you get clean meats, healthy fats, vegetables, and certain fruits on non-fast days, and you can structure your meals but best for you.

You may have lesser meals or snacks during the entire day or have a moderate lunch and dinner and quickly in the morning or after dinner during limited days. Concentrate once again on healthy fats, clean meats, and products. Apps can help you record food to don't go over 700 and record your calorie intake.

4. ADVANCED: 5-2 MEALS.

On this plan, five days a week, you're going to eat clean, but you won't eat anything for two days a week.

You can quickly eat clean food on Monday and Thursday, for example. Food will be the same as other fasting plans in these five days — healthy fats, clean meat, vegetables, and some fruit.

Remember that this plan is not intended for beginners and that you should talk with your doctor before actually starting a fasting procedure, particularly if you are under medicine or have a medical problem. Coffee drinkers are recommended to maintain a coffee supply in the morning and that all those who are fasting advanced stay properly hydrated.

- Monday: Fast.

- Tuesday: eat good fats, springs of clean meat, vegetables, and fruit.

- Wednesday: eat good fats, clean sources of meat, vegetables, and some fruit.

- Thursday: fast. Thursday: fast.

- Friday: eat healthy fats; eat clean meat and vegetables.

- Saturday: eat healthy fat, clean sources of meat, fruit, and vegetables

5. ADVANCED: EVERY OTHER DAY, SCHEDULE OR ALTERNATE FASTING.

Even if this plan is sophisticated, it is very straightforward.

You can eat healthy fats, clean meat, fruit, and vegetables every day, and then you can drink water, herbal tea, and a moderate quantity of black coffee or tea on your fasting days.

- Monday: eat clean meat, healthy fats, fruit, and vegetables.

- Tuesday: fast.

- Wednesday: eat good fats, clean sources of meat, vegetables, and some fruit.

- Thursday: fast.

- Friday: eat clean food, healthy fats, fruit, and vegetables.

- Saturday: fast.

- Sunday: eat clean meat sources, healthy fats, fruit, and vegetables.

You know precisely how to plan your meals when you start an intermittent fasting plan with this information in your hands. And although it may appear complicated at first, it'll feel like second nature and fit quite perfectly in your days once you get used to fasting. However, start working slowly and progressively to advanced plans.

It is also important to keep in mind that if intermittent fasting does not work for you, you may have some "off" days. Listen, if you have to eat outside your traditional window, it's all right. Just restart if you feel better.

8.2 Best Food and Recipes to break an intermittent fast

While Bullet Resistant coffee is a great way to break quickly, you can eat other foods to break your intermittent fasting duration.

To maximize IF benefits, most of your energy must be harvested from nutrient-dense foods while "feeding."

The selection of whole foods to make balanced foods will help you to get your body nutrients more powerful during fasts.

Breakfast with protein

Chicken, turkey, pork, seafood, beef, and eggs are favorite breaking proteins. You can eat mini quiches to make a fast first option for grab-and-heat.

Breakfast with healthy fats

As previously mentioned, coffee, noodles, grass-food butter, seeds, olive oil, nut butter, and coconut oil are all fastening options to eat quickly, and they are all great healthy food options.

Eat all of your veggies

It's always a great idea for you to break the fast with a gracious dose of veggies.

Eat a fruit portion

Fruits, fresh or frozen, are delicious micronutrient vessels. To sustain blood sugar levels, try to keep it in a single service. Try avoiding canned fruit or juice because the amounts of sugar per serving are concentrated.

Complex Carbohydrates to eat

Ideally, you want to reduce overall foods to break your speed, focusing on healthy fats and proteins. Skip the cereal bowl instead and eat an omelet or scrambled eggs.

Here are just a few deliciously simple recipes that provide a range of easy-to-prepare nutrients.

8.3 Easy Veggie Mini Quiches

Total Time: 25 mins.

Servings: 24 mini quiches

Ingredients

- Coconut oil (or any oil) 2 tsp.

- Grated packed green zucchini ¾ cup

- Packed grated carrots ¾ cup

- Green shallots (onions) 2, green tops trimmed off, white finely chopped (optional)

- Large eggs whisked 4

- Monterrey jack cheese grated ⅓ cup

- Salt ¼ tsp

Instructions

1. Preheat the oven at 180C and oil up your mini pan for cupcakes.

2. In a skillet, heat oil in medium heat. Add the zucchini, shallots, carrots, and cook. Stir for 5 to 7 minutes until the veggies soften up. Take away from heat and put aside to cool down near room temperature.

3. In a bigger bowl, combine veggies, grated cheese, eggs, and salt. Mix with a spoon into a mini muffin pan.

4. Bake for about 15-18 minutes. Let mini quiches cool down in the pan before removing them with a spatula or small knife carefully.

8.4 Roasted Veggies and Savory Oats Bowl

Total time: 35 mins

Servings: 4

Ingredients

- Bag-cubed butternut squash 16 ounce

- Brussels sprouts halved 8 ounces

- Olive oil 1 tbsp

- Salt divided 1 tsp

- Black pepper grounded 1 tsp

- Butter 1 tbsp

- Onion, coarsely chopped, ½ cup

- Old Fashioned Quaker Oats 2 cups

- Water 2 cups

- Sharp shredded Cheddar cheese ½ cup

- Eggs 4

- Crumbled cooked turkey bacon, two strips

Instructions

1. Preheat the oven up to 400F. Using the parchment line, a big baking sheet.

2. Mix the butternut squash, chopped onion, Brussels sprouts, olive oil, ½ tsp black pepper, and ½ tsp salt in a large bowl, toss to mix, and shift to the line of the baking sheet.

3. Bake till the veggies are golden brown or tender, which takes about 20-22 mins.

4. Melt the butter in a medium pot over medium heat while the vegetables roast. To toast the oats, add them to the pan and cook for about 30 seconds. Bring the water to a low boil, then reduce to low heat. Reduce to low heat and continue to cook for 8 to 10 mins, or until the oats hit a thick consistency, adding water as required. Season with the remaining pepper and salt and stir in the shredded cheese. Keep it warm.

5. Cook eggs yellow-side up or even over easy in a big greased nonstick pan.

6. Place oats in a bowl and top with vegetables, an egg, and bacon crumbles.

8.5 Spinach & Bacon Mini Quiches

Total time: 25 mins

Servings: mini quiches 24

Ingredients

- Eggs 6

- Milk 3 tbsp

- Finely chopped spinach ¾ cup

- Cheddar cheese, shredded 1 cup

- Bacon, cooked and chopped four strips

- Dash of pepper

Instructions

1. To 350 degrees Fahrenheit preheat the oven and butter up a 24 mini muffin pan.

2. In a big mixing bowl, whisk together the eggs and milk. Combine the chopped spinach, chopped bacon, shredded cheddar, and pepper in a mixing bowl. To combine all of the ingredients, give it a fast stir.

3. Uniformly distribute the egg mixture into the muffin pan cups.

4. Bake for 15-18 mins in a preheated oven.

5. When mini quiches are finished, set them aside to cool down in the pan before removing them with a spatula or small knife.

8.6 Cauliflower Shrimp Fried Rice

Total Time: 20 mins

Servings: 4

Ingredients

- Cauliflower one large head or cauliflower rice 6 cups

- Reduced sodium tamari, soy sauce, or coconut aminos, ¼ cup

- Honey 1 tbsp

- Grated fresh ginger ½ tsp or ground ginger ⅛ tsp.

- Red pepper flakes pinch

- Sesame oil 1 tbsp

- Green onions, chopped, greens separated from whites one bunch

- Frozen peas ½ cup

- Carrots, cubed ½ cup

- Beaten eggs, 3

- Shrimp, peeled, thawed, and deveined half lb.

Instructions

1. Put the cauliflower in a food processor and cut it up into pieces. Put aside after pulsing to chop till it resembles rice finely.

2. Combine San-J Tamari, honey, ginger, and red pepper flakes in a small bowl; set aside.

3. Heat sesame oil in a large wok or skillet over medium-high heat. Sauté for almost a min after adding the white portion of the onions. Stir in the frozen carrots and peas and heat up for about two mins. Transfer the vegetables to one end of the wok and pour in the beaten eggs. Cook eggs on one end of the pan until baked, turning the mixture around while it heats. Cook for about 2 mins, or until the shrimp have turned yellow.

4. Stir in the riced cauliflower until all is well mixed. Apply the Tamari sauce solution over the top, make sure it is uniformly dispersed, turn off the fire, add the green onions, and cover for a moment to soften.

Note

By removing the honey and replacing it with a honey substitute, you can make this recipe keto-friendly. You can significantly reduce the carbohydrate and sugar content by replacing the green peas and carrots with a higher fiber vegetable such as broccoli.

8.7 Mediterranean Chicken Farro Bowls

Since it's plain, quick, and fresh, this Mediterranean Chicken Farro Bowl is the ideal chicken bowl recipe for meal prep.

Total Time: 50 mins

Servings: 4

Ingredients

For the bowls

- Cooked bob's red mill farro 1 cup

- Water or stock 3 cups

- Salt ½ tsp

- Boneless chicken breasts 1 pound

- Olive oil three tbsp

- Zest of 1 lemon

- Lemon juice two tbsp

- Cloves garlic, grated 2

- Dried oregano 1 tsp

- Kosher salt ½ tsp

- Black pepper ¼ tsp

- Olive oil 1 tsp

- Cherry tomatoes, halved, 1 pint

- Chopped cucumber 2 cups

- Kalamata olives, sliced and pitted 1 cup

- Red onion, sliced ½ cup

- Tzatziki sauce 1 cup

- Crumbled feta cheese ½ cup

- Lemon wedges, to serve

- Fresh parsley and dill, for garnish

Tzatziki sauce

- Cucumber 1

- Garlic clove 1

- Cup plain yogurt 1

- Salt ½ tsp

- Lemon juice ½ tsp

- Dried dill ¼ tsp

Instructions

For the bowls

1. Drain and rinse the farro. In a jar, combine the farro, salt with enough stock or water to cover it. Bring to a boil, then reduce to medium-low heat and cook for thirty min. Any extra water should be drained.

2. For the chicken, prepare as follows: Combine chicken breasts, olive oil, lemon zest, lemon juice, garlic, oregano, salt, and pepper in a gallon zip pack. Marinate for four hours or a night in the refrigerator.

3. Heat the olive oil in a large skillet over medium-high heat, then add the chicken breasts and cook for seven min, flipping halfway through, until the temperature reached 165 degrees. Remove the marinade and discard it.

4. Remove the chicken from the pan and set it aside to cool for five min before slicing.

5. To make the Greek bowls, start by making a farro bed in the bowl bottom or meal Totaljar. Tzatziki sauce, feta cheese, sliced chicken, cucumber, olives, tomatoes, red onion, and tzatziki sauce. Serve with a garnish of parsley and dill and lemon wedges.

Tzatziki sauce

1. Insert a paper towel in the filter of a large bowl lined with a mesh strainer.

2. Grate the cucumber and garlic clove with a cheese grater, then strain to extract excess moisture.

3. Combine shredded cucumber, garlic, yogurt, salt, lemon juice, and dill in a medium mixing bowl. Combine all ingredients in a mixing bowl and chill for an hour before serving.

8.8 Super Greens Kale Salad with Sesame Ginger Dressing

This kale salad with sesame ginger dressing will quickly become a favorite of yours. This is one of the most delicious Asian-inspired salads you'll ever make.

Total time: 10 mins

Servings: 6–8

Ingredients

For the Salad:

- Chopped kale 6 cups (about one large head)

- Shredded red cabbage, 2 cups

- Shredded carrots 1 cup

- Shelled edamame 1 cup, heated if already frozen

- Finely sliced red onion half cup

- Sunflower seeds ¼ cup

Ingredients for the sesame ginger dressing

- Rice vinegar half cup

- Sesame seeds 3 tsp

- Soy sauce half cup

- Brown sugar 1 tsp

- Grated garlic clove only one

- Grated fresh ginger 2 tsp,

- Sesame oil 1 ½ tsp

Instructions

For the Kale Salad

1. In a big bowl, mix the red cabbage, layer kale, shredded carrots, red onion, shelled edamame, and sunflower seeds. Drizzle with Sesame Ginger Dressing and serve.

For the Sesame Ginger Dressing

1. To make the Sesame Ginger Dressing, add all of the ingredients to a mixing bowl.

2. Whisk together the dressing ingredients in a large mixing bowl. Refrigerate for up to one week in a glass container.

8.9 Sweet potato curry with spinach and chickpeas

This is a delightfully vegetarian curry having full flavor.

Total Time: 30mins

Servings: 6

Ingredients

- Chopped large, sweet onions half, or two scallions, finely sliced

- Canola oil 1-2 tsp

- Curry powder 2 tsp

- Cumin 1 tsp

- Cinnamon 1 tsp

- Washed, fresh spinach, coarsely chopped and stemmed 10 ounces

- Diced and peeled sweet potatoes 2 lbs.

- Chickpeas/cup water 14 1/2 ounce

- For garnish diced tomatoes, cup chopped cilantro 14 1/2 ounce

Instructions

1. You can cook the potatoes in any way you like.

2. One option is to peel, chop, and steam mine for about fifteen min in a veggie steamer.

3. Baking or boiling are also viable options.

4. Heat 1-2 tsp canola or veg oil over the moderate flame when sweet potatoes are cooking.

5. Add the onions and cook for 2-3 mins, or till they soften.

6. Stir in the curry powder, cumin, and cinnamon to uniformly cover the onions in spices.

7. Stir in the tomatoes and their juices, as well as the chickpeas.

8. Increase the heat to a heavy simmer for around a min or two after adding 12 cups of water.

9. Then, a few handfuls at a time, apply the fresh spinach, stirring to cover with the cooking liquid.

10. When all of the spinach has been applied to the pan, cover and cook for 3 mins, or until just wilted.

11. Stir the cooked potatoes into the liquid to coat them.

12. Cook for another 3-five min, or until all of the flavors are well blended.

13. Serve immediately after transferring to a serving dish and tossing it with fresh cilantro.

14. This dish goes well with brown rice or basmati rice.

8.10 Poached eggs & avocado toasts

Total Time: 15 mins

Servings: 4

Ingredients

- Eggs 4

- Ripe avocados 2

- Lemon juice 2 tsp

- Thick bread four slices

- Grated cheese 1 cup

- Salt and black pepper freshly ground

- Butter 4 tsp

Instructions

1. Using your favorite tool to poach eggs.

2. Meanwhile, strip the stones from the avocados and cut them in half.

3. Scoop the flesh into a bowl with a spoon, then add the lime or lemon juice, salt, and pepper.

4. Using a fork, mash the potatoes roughly.

5. Butter the toast and spread it with butter.

6. Top each piece of buttered toast with the avocado mixture and a poached egg.

7. Serve immediately with a sprinkle of grated cheese.

8. With grilled or fresh tomato halves on the side, these are both delicious.

8.11 Vegan fried 'fish' tacos

Total Time: 50 mins

Servings: 8 small tacos

Ingredients

- Silken tofu 14 ounces

- Panko breadcrumbs 2 cups

- Plain flour ½ cup

- Salt ½ tsp

- Smoked paprika 1 tsp

- Cayenne pepper half tsp

- Ground cumin 1 tsp

- Non-dairy milk ½ cup

- Vegetable oil, for frying ¼

- Head cabbage, shredded

- Ripe avocado 1

- Small tortillas 8

- Vegan mayonnaise, to serve

- Pickled onion

- Red onion, finely sliced, peeled, 1

- Apple cider vinegar ¼ cup

- Sugar 1 tsp

Instructions

1. To remove excess moisture, pat the tofu with a few pieces of kitchen paper. Split the tofu into ragged 1-inch chunks with a knife – let them be imperfect rather than cubes, so they look better.

2. In a large shallow bowl, combine the breadcrumbs.

3. In a separate wide shallow bowl, combine the flour, smoked paprika, salt, smoked paprika, cayenne, and cumin.

4. In a third-wide shallow bowl, pour the milk.

5. Toss the tofu chunks in the flour, then the milk, then the breadcrumbs, and place them on a baking sheet.

6. Fill a thick frying pan with vegetable oil to a depth of half an inch. Place over medium heat and allow the oil to heat up – if a breadcrumb begins to bubble and brown, the oil is ready. Fry small pieces of breaded tofu until golden underneath, then flip and finish cooking until golden all over. To drain, place on a baking sheet covered with kitchen paper. Rep with the rest of the tofu.

7. To make the pickled onion, combine the following ingredients in a small bowl.

8. In a small pot, heat the apple cider vinegar, salt, and sugar until steaming. Add the vinegar over the thinly chopped red onion in a jar or bowl. Allow it to soften and turn pink for at least thirty min.

9. Serve the hot fried tofu with pickled onion, vegan mayo, avocado, and shredded **cabbage in warmed tortillas.**

8.12 Sweet potato and black bean burrito

Total Time: 1 hr. 5 mins

Servings: 8 to 12 portions

Ingredients

- Cubed, peeled sweet potatoes 5 cups

- Salt half tsp

- Other vegetable oil or broth 2 tsp

- Diced onions 3 1/2 cups

- Garlic cloves, minced 4

- Minced green chili pepper (fresh) 1 tsp

- Ground cumin 4 tsp

- Ground coriander 4 tsp

- Black beans cooked (three cans of 15-ounce, drained) 4 1/2 cups

- Cilantro leaf lightly packed 2/3 cup

- Fresh lemon juice 2 tsp

- Flour tortillas (10 inches) 12

- Fresh salsa

Instructions

1. Preheat oven to 350 degrees Fahrenheit.

2. In a medium saucepan, combine the sweet potatoes, salt, and enough water to cover them.

3. Cover and insert in a boil, then reduce to low heat and cook until the vegetables are tender for about 10 mins.

4. Drain the water and set it aside.

5. Heat the oil in a medium saucepan or skillet and bring the garlic, onions, and chili, whereas the potatoes are cooking.

6. Cover and cook on low heat, with the occasional stir, for about 7 mins, or until the onions are tender.

7. Cook, frequently stirring, for another 2 to 3 mins after adding the cumin and coriander.

8. Take the pan off the flame and set it aside.

9. Puree the black beans, salt, cilantro, cooked sweet potatoes, and lemon juice in a food processor until smooth (or mash the ingredients in a large bowl by hand).

10. Add the cooked spices and onions to the sweet potato mixture in a large mixing bowl.

11. A big baking dish should be lightly oiled.

12. Fill each tortilla with about 2/3-3/4 cup of filling; after rolling, place it seam side down in the baking dish.

13. Bake for 30 mins, or until piping hot, covered tightly with foil.

14. **Serve with salsa on top.**

8.13 Perfect cauliflower pizza crust

Total Time: 1hr 10mins

Servings: 4

Ingredients

- Raw cauliflower (riced) 4 cups or one medium cauliflower head

- Egg, beaten 1

- Chevre cheese or other soft cheese 1 cup

- Dried oregano 1 tsp

- Pinch salt 1

Instruction

1. Preheat the oven to 400 degrees Fahrenheit.

2. To make cauliflower rice, in a food processor, place the raw cauliflower florets batches till a texture like rice is achieved.

3. Bring a pot of water to a boil with just over an inch of water in it. Cook for around 4-5 mins after adding the "rice" and covering it. Drain into a strainer with a fine mesh.

4. Once the rice has been strained, shift it to a tidy, thin dishtowel. Wiggle all the extra moisture out of the steamed rice by wrapping it in a dishtowel, twisting it up. It's incredible how much extra moisture will be released, resulting in a nice, dry pizza crust.

5. Combine the beaten egg, strained rice, spices, and goat cheese in a large mixing bowl. (Do not be afraid to mix it with your hands; thoroughly mix it.) It won't be like any other pizza dough you've ever seen, but don't worry; it'll hold together.

6. Place the dough on a baking sheet that has been covered with parchment paper. Keep the dough about 3/8" thick, and allow the edges a little too higher for a "crust" effect, if you like. (It must be propped with parchment paper; otherwise, it'll stick.)

7. Bake at 400 degrees F for 35-40 mins, or until the crust is firm and golden brown.

8. Now is the time to add all of your favorite toppings, including cheese, sausage, and any other ingredients you desire. Restore the pizza to the oven and bake for another 5-10 mins, or until cheese is melted and bubbling.

9. Slice and serve right away.

8.14 Cobb salad with brown derby dressing

Total time: 30 mins

Servings: 2

Ingredients

- Head iceberg lettuce ½

- Bunch watercress ½

- Bunch chicory lettuce 1

- Head romaine lettuce 1/2

- Medium tomatoes (seeded and skinned) 2

- Smoked turkey breast half lb.

- Slices crisp bacon 6

- Avocado, sliced in half, peeled and seeded 1

- Hardboiled eggs 3

- Chives, finely chopped 2 tsp

- Crumbled blue cheese, ½ cup

Dressing

- Water 2 tsp

- Sugar 1/8 tsp

- Kosher salt ¾ tsp

- Worcestershire sauce half tsp

- Balsamic vinegar 2 tsp

- Fresh lemon juice 1 tsp

- Fresh grounded black pepper 1/2 tsp

- Dijon mustard 1/8 tsp

- Olive oil 2 tsp

- Cloves garlic, finely minced 2

Instructions

1. Finely chop all of the greens (almost minced).

2. In a cold salad bowl, arrange in rows.

3. Break the tomatoes in two, remove the seeds, and chop finely.

4. The ham, avocado, eggs, and bacon should all be finely diced.

5. Arrange all of the ingredients in rows around the lettuces, including the blue cheese.

6. Lastly, add the chives.

7. Present in this manner at the table, then swirl with the dressing before serving in cold salad bowls.

8. Serve with a side of freshly baked French bread.

9. TO MAKE THE DRESSING: In a blender, combine all of the ingredients, except the olive oil, and blend until smooth.

10. Slowly drizzle in the oil when the unit is working, and thoroughly blend.

11. Keep refrigerated until ready to use.

Note:

Keep this dish chilled and eat it as cold as possible.

8.15 Chicken coconut curry along with broccoli rice (Keto)

Total time: 45 mins.

Servings: 4-6

Ingredients

- Macadamia oil 2 tsp

- Lilydale chicken thigh (free-range), pieces cut into the length of 3cm, 600g

- Brown onion sliced 1

- Garlic cloves, crushed 2

- Thinly grated fresh ginger 2

- Long red chilies, thinly chopped, and extra sliced for serving 2

- Turmeric ½ tsp

- Brown mustard seeds 2 tsp

- Ground cumin 2 tsp

- Ground coriander 1 tsp

- Can coconut cream 400ml

- Broccoli, chopped 500g

- Lime juice, for taste

- Fish sauce, for taste

- Baby spinach leaves 100g

Instructions

1. In a big saucepan or wok, heat half the oil over high heat. Cook, stirring periodically, for 2-3 min or until the chicken is browned. Place on a plate to cool. Carry on with the rest of the chicken.

2. In the same pan, add the rest of the oil and the onion. Cook for 3-4 mins, stirring occasionally, or until softened. Turmeric, garlic, chili, ginger, mustard seeds, coriander, and cumin should all be added at this stage. Cook for 2 mins, stirring occasionally, or till aromatic. Combine the coconut cream with chicken in a mixing bowl. Get the water to a boil. Lower the heat and partly cover. Cook for 20 mins, or until chicken is cooked through.

3. Meanwhile, in a food processor, finely chop the broccoli until it resembles rice, working in batches if required. In a

big microwave-safe bowl, put the broccoli. Microwave for 2-3 min on HIGH until it is just tender.

4. Remove the curry from the heat and season to taste with fish sauce and lime juice. Serve with broccoli rice and a sprinkling of spinach and extra chili.

8.16 Healthy tuna mornay

Total time: 30 min

Servings: 6

Try this healthy version of classic tuna pasta bake for low-calorie comfort food.

Ingredients

- Olive oil 1 tsp

- Onion, finely chopped 1

- Celery sticks, thinly chopped 2

- Large carrot, finely chopped, peeled 1

- zucchini, thinly sliced 2

- Green beans, cut into lengths of 1 cm 200g

- Olive oil spread 1 1/2 tsp

- Plain flour 2 tsp

- Reduced-fat milk 500ml (2 cups)

- Can tuna of spring water, flaked, drained 425g

- Grated parmesan 40g (1/2 cup)

- Cooked brown rice 270g (2 cups)

- Baby spinach leaves 120g

- To serve, mixed salad leaves

Instructions

1. Preheat the oven to 190 degrees /170 degrees Fahrenheit if using a fan-forced oven. Using a light spray of oil, lightly coat a 2L ovenproof baking dish.

2. In a wide saucepan over medium heat, heat the oil. Cook, occasionally stirring, for 5 mins or till the onion, celery, and carrot are softened. Cook, stirring regularly, for 2 mins, or until the zucchini and beans are just tender. Place the vegetables in a mixing bowl.

3. Return to the same pan over medium heat and melt the spread. Stir in the flour until it is well mixed. Slowly drizzle in the milk, stirring continuously, until smooth and well mixed. Bring to a boil, reduce to low heat, and continue to stir continuously until the sauce thickens. Combine the vegetables, tuna, and half of the parmesan cheese in a mixing bowl. It's that time of year.

4. Cover the bottom of the baking dish with rice. The spinach comes first, followed by the tuna mixture. Finish with the

rest of the parmesan cheese. Cook for 20 mins, or until golden brown and bubbly. Until serving with salad leaves, set aside for 5 mins.

Notes

To make a dairy-free version, substitute the lowered fat milk with reduced-fat soy milk and half cup grated Cheese with parmesan.

8.17 Southern-style sweet potato salad

Total Time: 40 mins

Servings 6

Ingredients

- Large sweet potatoes, thickly sliced, halved lengthways, 2

- Olive oil 1 tbsp

- Cajun seasoning 1 tbsp

- Corn cob, silk and husk removed 1

- Buttermilk 1/3 cup (80ml)

- Whole-egg mayonnaise 1/4 cup (75g)

- Lime juice 1 tbsp

- Finely chopped coriander 1/4 cup

- Avocado, cut in the shape of wedges (thin), stoned, and peeled 1

- Red capsicum, seeded, finely sliced 1

- Red onion, finely sliced 1

- Coriander sprigs 1/2 cup

Instructions

1. Potato, charred corn, creamy avocado, and a zingy buttermilk dressing are mixed.

2. Preheat the oven to 200 degrees Celsius. Using the baking paper, line a baking tray. In a large mixing bowl, add the sweet potato, oil, and Cajun seasoning. Arrange on a lined tray in a single sheet. Bake for 30 mins, or till sweet potato is tender, turning once.

3. Meanwhile, preheat a medium-hot barbecue grill or chargrill. Cook for 10 mins, turning periodically or until slightly charred and tender. Allow cooling before serving. To release the kernels, chop down the part of the corn with a knife.

4. In a small mixing bowl, add the buttermilk, lime juice, chopped coriander, and mayonnaise.

5. In a big mixing bowl, combine sweet potato, avocado, capsicum, corn, onion, and coriander sprigs. Drizzle the buttermilk dressing over the salad and toss gently to mix. Place on a serving platter and serve.

8.18 Asian Noodles with Chicken

Total Time: 13 mins

Servings: 2

Ingredients

- Bundle of dried fine egg noodles 1

- Chicken breast sliced in the shape of ribbons with the grain of meat 200 g

- Ginger finely chopped and peeled 1 piece

- Cloves garlic finely chopped and peeled 2

- Handful green beans tailed and topped

- Chinese leaf or similar thinly shredded 100 g

- Courgettes sliced in the form of batons 150 g

- Red chili de-seeded and thinly sliced 1

- Low salt soy 2 tsp

- Sunflower or sesame oil 1 tsp

- Fresh coriander 1 handful

- Chicken or vegetable stock 300 ml

- Coconut cream 1 tsp

Instructions

1. In a wok, heat the oil and cook the shallot, garlic, ginger, and chili for about a min.

2. The chicken should now be added and sealed on all sides.

3. Cook for about a min after adding the courgette batons.

4. Stir in the remaining vegetables for a min.

5. Stir in the soy sauce and stock, and then add the noodles.

6. Cook till the noodles are soft (about 3 mins), then add the coriander and, if using, the coconut cream.

7. Serve with the rest of the coriander leaves on top.

8.19 Chili Beef Stir Fry

Total Time: 10 mins

Servings: 1

Ingredients

- Fillet steak or lean cut 50g

- Continental Spring Onion 1 (or two smaller ones)

- Broccoli 100 g

- Courgettes 100 g

- Chinese Cabbage or pak choi 100 g

- Clove Garlic crushed 1

- Red Chili seeded and finely chopped 1/2

- Root Ginger finely chopped and peeled 1 piece

- Chinese rice wine vinegar 1 tsp

- Light Soy 1 tsp

- Sunflower or Sesame oil 1 tsp

Instructions

1. Combine the chili, ginger, rice, soy sauce, garlic, and wine vinegar in a mixing bowl.

2. Finely slice the beef against the grain, then toss it in the soy mixture.

3. Slice the spring onion after trimming it. Keep the green leaves and white bulbs apart.

4. Slice all of the vegetables into smallish bits.

5. In a wok, heat the oil until it is barely smoking. Drain the beef and apply it to the oil with white sections of the spring onion and Chinese cabbage, reserving the soy mixture. For a min, cook

6. Add the Chinese cabbage and broccoli and cook for a few mins more, stirring continuously, until the vegetables are cooked but still crunchy.

7. Pour in the rest of the soy and chili mixture and mix well.

8. Garnish with the green sections of the onion (spring) and a small amount of boiled rice.

8.20 Tomato Soup with Roasted Garlic and Basil

Total Time: 1 hr. 35 mins

Servings: 6

Ingredients

- Ripe Tomatoes 1 kg (mixture of vine tomatoes, plum tomatoes, and cherry tomatoes)

- Bulb Garlic 1

- Stick Celery 1

- Small Carrot 1

- Banana Shallots 2

- Balsamic Vinegar NB ½ - 1 tsp (in case of strong vinegar, reduce the amount)

- Chopped handful Basil Stems 1, leaves kept for garnish

- Olive Oil 1 tsp

- Sugar 1 tsp

- Stock Marigold 500 ml or fresh chicken stock

Instructions

1. Place the tomatoes cut side up on a baking tray after cutting them in half lengthwise. Season with salt and pepper, then drizzle with a small amount of olive oil, reserving around a tsp. Remove the head of the garlic bulb and cover it in tinfoil.

2. To 190°C, preheat the oven and bake the tomatoes and garlic bulb for about an hour, or until the tomatoes are soft and the edges are beginning to char.

3. Place the celery, carrot, and shallot in a large stockpot with the remaining oil and finely diced celery, carrot, and shallot. Cook for 8-10 mins, or until the mixture begins to soften, over low heat. Remove from the heat and set aside until the tomatoes are ready.

4. Toss the mixed vegetables with the tomatoes and all of their juices. Squeeze all of the softened garlic into a bowl with a fork, discarding the skin and base. Toss the tomato mixture with the garlic paste. Connect the basil stems to the mix.

5. Bring to a boil with the stock. Until blending with a stick blender, cook for about 20 mins, before rechecking the seasoning, substitute half of the balsamic. Add a tsp or two of sugar, salt, and pepper to taste, and the rest of the balsamic vinegar.

6. Serve hot or cold with croutons, creme fraiche, Greek yogurt, or crispy garlic.

8.21 Slimline Livorno Fish Stew

Total Time: 35 mins

Servings: 2

Ingredients

- Mussels 4

- Squid Tube 1

- Whitefish (hake) 150 g

- Green Prawns 4

- Red Chili half

- Cloves Garlic 2

- Stick Celery 1

- Tomatoes (preferably plum) 4

- Rustic Bread Roll 1

- Handful leaves parsley (Flat) 1

- Olive oil 1 tsp

- Shallot 1

- Stock 100ml or dry white wine

Instructions

1. Halve the tomatoes, then grate the flesh and remove the skins.

2. Roughly chop the onion, celery, garlic, and chili, then process until finely diced in a food processor (or chop by hand)

3. Cook the chopped veggies in olive oil for around 5-10 mins, stirring occasionally.

4. Combine the tomato mixture, the majority of the parsley, and the stock or wine in a mixing bowl. Reduce the temperature for another 15 mins.

5. Slice the squid and chop white fish into bite-sized chunks.

6. Cook for 5 mins with the white fish, squid, and prawns in the tomato mixture.

7. Place the mussels in a microwave-safe dish with a small amount of water. Microwave the mussels for 3-4 mins, discarding those and do not open.

8. Add the mussels to the stew

9. If using bread, toast it on the grill in a few mins until golden.

10. Toss the bread into the bottoms of flattish bowls before spooning the stew on top.

11. Serve garnished with parsley.

8.22 Courgetti with Aubergine and Tuna

Total time: 35 mins

Servings: 2

Ingredients

- Medium courgette 2

- Medium aubergine 1

- Tuna or swordfish 180 g

- Medium tomatoes (ripen) 2

- Clove garlic crushed 1

- Handful fresh mint 1

- Handful basil or parsley 1

- Lemon 1 or white wine

- Olive oil 2 tsp

Instructions

1. Cut the aubergine in two lengthwise and steam for 20 mins over boiling water until tender.

2. Allow it to cool slightly before chopping into chunks and tossing the mint into the aubergine.

3. Cut the tops and tails from the courgettes, then slice them into ribbons with a potato peeler.

4. Chop the tomato and fish (if using fresh) into small pieces.

5. In a separate pan, soften the garlic, cover the tuna, stir in the tomato with aubergine, and set aside while the courgettes cook.

6. Heat a tsp of olive oil in a large nonstick frying pan, then carefully soften the courgettes on just moderate heat until they start to turn translucent.

7. Toss in the sauce, season to taste with salt, pepper, and lemon juice, and toss in the basil leaves.

8. Serve.

8.23 Hake on Braised Potatoes with Garlic, Tomato, and Olives

Total Time: 20 mins

Servings: 2

Ingredients

Fish

- Hake Steaks 2

- Olive Oil 1 tsp

- cloves garlic thinly Sliced 4

- Potatoes sliced and Peeled 250 g

- Shallots finely chopped 2

- Chicken Stock 200ml

- Tomatoes Skinned 150 g

- Parley Chopped 1 tsp

- Kalamata Olives 8

Caramelized Garlic

- Garlic Cloves chopped 100 g

- Olive oil 2 tsp

Instructions

Caramelized Garlic

1. In a small pan, combine olive oil and garlic and cook over low heat for 15-20 mins, stirring regularly and mixing it up as it softens.

2. Remove it from the oven until it's finished, slightly caramelized, and smooth, and set it aside to cool.

Fish

1. Set aside the fish steaks after seasoning them with salt.

2. In an ovenproof skillet, heat the remaining olive oil and soften the garlic and shallots for around 10 mins.

3. Bring skinned tomatoes and cook for about 3 mins, or until softened and mashed down with a fork.

4. Pour in the stock and carry to a gentle simmer.

5. Cover and add the potatoes. Cook for 15-20 mins on the stovetop or until the potatoes are only tender.

6. For 2 mins, Grill the fish on either side.

7. Carefully place the fish on top of the baste and potatoes with a light sauce. Toss in the olives.

8. Return to the oven for another 10 mins or until the fish is thoroughly cooked.

9. Garnish each serving with half a tsp of caramelized garlic and 1/2 tsp. of chopped parsley. The leftover garlic can be kept for a few days in the fridge in an airtight bag.

Chapter 9: Myths of Intermittent Fasting

9.1   Myth 1: When Intermittent Fasting, You Can't Focus.

Consider the very last time we were really hungry. It wasn't likely your best zen moment.

You do not feel this "hangry" condition if you practice intermittent fasting regularly. Your hunger hormones will regulate until your cells have adapted to the use of body fat for energy. Ketones are small molecules that provide clean, usable energy to your brain as you burn body fat. It's been shown that promoting ketosis increases attention, concentration, and focus for older adults.

9.2   Myth 2: Intermittent Fasting Causes the Metabolism to Decrease.

Some people believe that fasting causes the resting metabolic rate to decrease. In other words, intermittent fasting makes you burn lesser calories at rest. The fear is that you will gain weight like a three-toed sloth if you resume regular eating habits. That is what happens on calorie-restricted diets, which require you to consume 50 to 85 percent of calories your body regularly needs for a long time. Your body adjusts to the reduced energy intake and can do so for years. You have probably observed calorie restriction in effect on The Biggest Loser. While the contestants lose weight, they almost always regain it. The show never mentions that aspect, which is inconvenient for viewers.

Is intermittent fasting the same as regular fasting? It does not seem to be the case. Non-obese people who observed alternate-day fasting retained a regular metabolic rate again for the majority of three weeks, even while burning more fat, according to a 2005 report study in the American Journal for Clinical Nutrition.

9.3 Myth 3: Everyone Can use it

Intermittent fasting is all the rage these days. In certain cases, it is sold as being helpful to all, all of the time. While fasting is generally healthy and safe for the majority of people, some groups should avoid it. The following are some of these groups: kids, pregnant and nursing women, and underweight people. The groups as mentioned above need more food, not lesser. Fasting's possible advantages are outweighed by the chance of nutrient deficiency. Those with high blood sugar must exercise caution as well. Fasting may be beneficial for this population, but medical supervision is needed to avoid extremely low blood sugar (hypoglycemia).

9.4 Myth 4: When Intermittent Fasting, you should Not Drink Water

Some religious fasts, such as Ramadan fasting, limit both food and water. Unrelated to this, various reports have emerged claiming that no-water fasts were beneficial to one's wellbeing. Due to the diuretic effect of fasting, restricting water may lead to disastrous dehydration. That's why, when supervising patients on therapeutic fasts, doctors pay careful attention to fluid intake. Electrolytes, including sodium and potassium, energetically ripped out during fasting, are often monitored by doctors. What's the takeaway? During a fast, drink plenty of water and take potassium and sodium supplements if the fast lasts longer than 13 or 15 hours.

9.5 Myth 5: No matter what, you'll lose weight.

Contrary to common belief, intermittent fasting, even fasting in particular, does not necessarily result in weight loss. This type of mindset is a common misconception whenever it comes to these types of dieting. No know how old you've been fasting. The chances of surviving are slim to nil if you're breaking this with fries, burgers, and candy. Each fasting day should never be deemed a cheat day in order and for the diet to function.

Myth: When you break your fast, you can consume as much as you'd like.

Intermittent fasting, as with every other diet, is just starting a healthier way of life. Unfortunately, many people believe that they can resume their usual eating habits once their fast is over. This is in direct opposition to all of them working hard. The most interesting thing to remember when it applies to I.F. is to skip breakfast when you've broken the fast. You would have lost your fasting time if you fasted all day before dinner and only ate dinner the size of breakfast/lunch/dinner.

9.6 Myth 6: Intermittent Fasting will make you incredibly safe and fit.

When combined with good practice and exercise, intermittent fasting will lead to weight loss. However, anyone adopting the diet should be mindful that it is not a successful way of losing weight independently. There is no one-size-fits-all solution. Don't take health and happiness for granted; they're things you'd work hard to keep in your life. Fasting won't give you the ideal body overnight, and even if you lose the weight, you'll have had to keep it off with healthy habits like eating better and exercising regularly.

Myth 8: Intermittent Fasting will make you incredibly safe and fit.

In long-term clinical trials, participants in the fasting groups showed no signs of hunger or dietary deficiency. The performance of the diets should be prioritized when breaking the fast. Finally, since chubby vitamins become readily accessible when absorbed through circulation from fat stores, nutritional shortages can be avoided by restricting refined, nutrient-poor diets and growing nutrient-dense, unprocessed foods.

9.7 Myth 7: Intermittent Fasting is nothing more than starvation.

Fasting is a conscious act in which one refrains from feeding for a specified period. True starvation happens when food is unavailable for an unknown period, and the person has little control over the situation. When people fast, their endogenous insulin levels decrease, meaning that they are not hungry and get regular calories through fat stores.

9.8 Myth 8: The most significant food of the day will be breakfast.

Breakfast is needed to give you the extra boost you need to get your day started. If you don't eat first thing every morning, your body will respond by raising adrenaline (growth hormone) and cortisol levels, causing the liver to produce glucose, giving you the energy you need to get through the day. As a consequence, breakfast isn't as important as it once was. Breakfast is typically associated with eating first thing in the morning. It is much more socially acceptable to acknowledge that it doesn't matter whenever the phrase is decomposed (breakfast) if one breaks the overnight soon.

9.9 Myth 9: Intermittent Fasting Causes Overreacting

You'll be hungry after a short. Many people believe that this hunger would lead to overeating. The proof, on the other hand, refutes this concern. Ad libitum feeding refers to the process of allowing participants to consume as much as they want during a fasting study. They eat to their hearts' content and still lose weight. Many intermittent fasting protocols would cause you to eat less rather than more. As a result of the moderate calorie restriction, you'll lose weight gradually without slowing down your metabolism.

9.10 Myth 10: If You Fast, You Will Not Gain Muscle.

Fasting does not seem to be the only way to gain muscle mass. Do you still need to pounds protein shakes? Protein is necessary, but it is not needed all of the time. In one 2019 report, for example, healthy women who fasted 16/8 gained the same amount of strength and muscle as women who ate on a more traditional schedule. Here's the deal: In times of shortage, the body works overtime to conserve muscle. When you fast, your body fat (rather than muscle) is used to meet your energy needs.

Consider this: if we burned across muscle throughout a fast, our forefathers would have been unable to hunt!

9.11 Myth 11: Lack of Energy Is Caused by intermittent fasting

Food is a source of energy. Would your energy levels fall if you don't have them?

Yes, eventually. When the fast intermittently, though, your cells switch to a different source of energy: body fat. There's plenty of it to go around. That's right. Even a thin person (e.g., 150 pounds of 10% body fat) has significant fat reserves to meet energy demands when fasting. Fifteen pounds of fat equals over 60,000 calories for energy if you do the math! In reality, many people claim that exercising while fasted gives them more energy. After a big meal, blood is redirected away from muscles and into digestive organs, making sense.

Chapter 10: Remedies for coping up with the drawbacks of fasting

Although the advantages of intermittent fasting greatly outweigh the disadvantages, a few minor aggravating adverse effects, one of which is intermittent fasting (IF) headache. You have probably had a fasting headache if you've ever been without food for an extended time (much longer than the body is used to). On your fast day or during the fasting window, headaches are more likely to occur for the following reasons:

- Hypoglycemia (Low blood sugar levels)

- Dehydration

- Electrolyte Deficiency

- Caffeine Withdrawal

On the plus side, there are many ways to handle and minimize these Disadvantages so that you do not have to avoid fasting and keep going before your goal-feeding window arrives. Below is an overview of each of these factors and treatments that have helped me and others.

The Causes will eventually fade away as you move through your fasting journey.

10.1 Hypoglycemia

When the body's sugar, glucose level falls below 70mg/dL, hypoglycemia occurs. Headaches, irritability, fatigue, dizziness, shakiness, plus hunger are all symptoms of low glucose. If you eat a high-sugar meal before the fasting window begins, you may experience a rapid rise of blood sugar followed by a rapid drop, resulting in a headache.

Remedy

Before beginning your fasting time, avoid carbs with such a high glycemic index (GI). If you want to eat high-GI carbs, eat them in the middle during your feeding window, and low-GI carbs at the end during your fasting period. Low GI carbs cause the blood sugar levels to fluctuate much less, which can help minimize the huge glucose spikes that cause intermittent fasting headaches.

10.2 Dehydration

Intermittent fasting headaches may be caused by dehydration. Water can make up 50-65 percent of the average human body composition. This means that, in addition to oxygen, consuming water is important. Perhaps more so, the brain is composed of 75% water, and a lack of water will cause your brain to contract or shrink momentarily due to fluid loss, resulting in dehydration headaches. This pain is caused by your brain moving away from your skull, according to Medical News Today. Headaches are one of the most common symptoms of dehydration. There are some other symptoms like:

- dark-colored urine

- reduced urination

- extreme thirst

- confusion

- dizziness

- fatigue

- dry, sticky mouth

Remedy

So, the only solution would be to drink water. You should drink at least 12 gallons of water a day, and I suggest at least one gallon if you are doing strenuous workouts.

10.3 Electrolyte Deficiency

Electrolyte imbalances are another cause of intermittent fasting headaches. Drinking electrolyte-rich water will help you stick to your quick. Electrolytes are chemical components of the body needed for various physiological functions, including muscular contractions, nerve impulses, heart function, and brain function, to name a few. Sodium, magnesium, also potassium are the three main electrolytes the body needs throughout intermittent fasting. Intermittent fasting aims to reduce insulin levels to use fat reserves for energy and lose weight. When you lower your insulin levels, your body retains less sodium and water, contributing to electrolyte imbalances. The following are some of the most common symptoms of electrolyte deficiency:

- aches and pains

- Feeling dizzy

- Confusion

- Fatigue

- Muscle spasms

- Heart pounding

This is why electrolytes must be consumed when fasting.

Remedy

We give you the general rule of thumb for eating enough sodium and keep the electrolytes balanced when fasting.

Thumb's rule:

Get at least 2000 mg of sodium per day (one to two tsp of salt). Shoot for 4000-7000 mg-s if you are physically active either sweat a lot (2-3 tsp of salt). "Mixed with water." suggests using

Himalayan salt instead of standard table salt in your water. The health benefits of Himalayan salt are well-known. Here are some amazing drink recipes that help remedy intermittent fasting headaches and ensure you get all of the appropriate chemicals you need during your fast.

Himalayan salt and Lemon are combined in this drink to relieve headaches in minutes. This salt plus lemon drink helps to improve your immune function, boost stamina, restore alkaline balance in your body, and raise serotonin levels, in addition to resolving electrolyte imbalances.

10.4 Caffeine Withdrawal

Intermittent fasting headaches are often caused by caffeine withdrawal. When you are used to drinking multiple cups of tea and coffee every day and suddenly quit, your body may not like it, and you may experience headaches as a result.

Remedy

Caffeine is good for you! Your fast will not be broken by coffee or tea. Coffee and tea should be consumed because they help increase the pace at which we burn body fat and leave you feeling satiated. GABA (Gamma-aminobutyric acid) is a chemical found in black coffee that helps you feel healthy and relaxed. Green tea, in particular, contains a chemical named epigallocatechin - 3- gallate (EGCG), which aids in the management of your fast as well as the reduction of hunger. So, when you are hungry, grab that cup of green tea!

It is recommended that you should not use creamers or sugar in your tea or coffee. These items will break your fast, which you do not want to happen. You just do not want to consume too much caffeine. Caffeine in excess may have a harmful impact by revving up your adrenals and increasing your cortisol levels. Cortisol levels rising could lead to insulin levels rising, and intermittent fasting would aim to maintain insulin levels low so that fat stores can be activated for energy. So do not squander it by overindulging in coffee.

Chapter 11: Intermittent Fasting Rules

Follow these ten guidelines to ensure you are on the right track, whether you're new to intermittent fasting and if you've been doing it for a while and it's not working out for you.

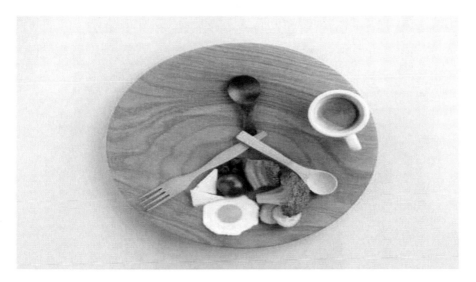

11.1 Begin gradually: Try Crescendo Fasting.

Crescendo fasting entails only fasting several days a week rather than every day. You will gradually introduce the body to fasting this way, ensuring that you stay committed to it.

The commonly used method would be to fast over 12 – 16 hours twice or three times a week on alternating days. The "fasting window" for this form of fasting is 12-16 hours, and the "feeding window" is 8-12 hours. This method of fasting is a lot less difficult to adopt. Simply skipping breakfast is a simple way to get started.

When fasting becomes approached in this manner, you will lose more weight while still gaining a lot of energy. In addition, crescendo fasting becomes safer, more natural, and puts the body under less stress.

11.2 Portion Sizes Should Be Restricted

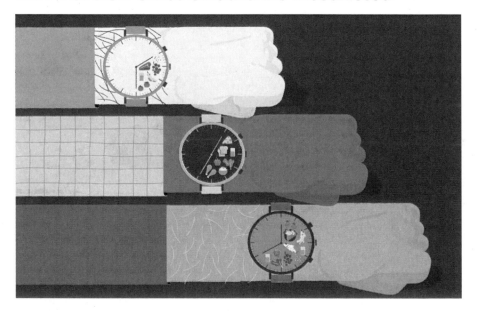

What would you do if you have already limited your meals to 12 hours per day but aren't seeing any results? Consider limiting the amount of food you eat. To see the full benefits of intermittent fasting, most experts recommend limiting the daily food consumption to two meals a day.

This rule is especially important for people who are overweight or obese since they tend to overeat whenever they break or finish their fast. So, if you want to lose weight quickly, pay attention to your portion sizes and begin calorie restriction.

11.3 Choose an Appropriate Eating Window

Keep in mind that everyone's needs and routines are different, and there is no one-size-fits-all eating window. People who exercise every morning tend to go to bed hungry, while others cannot sleep without a proper meal.

So, rather than blindly following others, try creating your schedule. If you prefer to eat dinner with your mates, you can shift your mealtime from 12 to 8 p.m. However, if you cannot start a day with no breakfast, this same eating window could be from 8 a.m. to 4 p.m.

Do whatever works the best for you, as well as follow it religiously.

11.4 Experiment with a 12-hour feeding window.

Although some people say that a 24-hour fast is ideal for them, experts advise against taking such a drastic approach. It is usually recommended to refrain from fasting for longer periods on an even regular basis.

What is the reason for this?

According to the experts, limiting your food intake for six hours regularly may raise the risk for gallstone formation. This raises the risk of complications, including the need for gallbladder removal.

Fasting for extended periods has also been shown in studies to raise the risk for gallstone development in women, regardless of their weight. [two]

Maintaining a 12-hour feeding window (no or less than 8 hours) is usually considered healthy and can result in successful fat loss.

11.5 Eat Protein-Rich Foods

Alternate-day fasting has several negative consequences, including a significant impact on the body muscles, leading to muscle wasting. To compensate, increase the amount of protein throughout your meals.

Protein-rich meals may not only help you retain muscle mass, but they can also help you curb your appetite. Good foods to be included in your daily meals include chicken, eggs, oats, as well as nuts.

11.6 Drink Lots of Water

It is important to remember to drink water during the day. During your fasting period, please ensure you drink plenty of water. This is especially significant for people who have only recently begun to practice intermittent fasting.

You should drink black coffee, unsweetened tea in addition to water. Milk and sweeteners should not be added to your drinks because they can break your fast.

11.7 Do not Force Yourself to Workout Fasted

Many people enjoy fasted workouts. In a fasted state, they feel more energized and devote more time to their training sessions. This, however, may not be what that everybody can do. Some people like to change their eating window so that they can eat before exercising. This is completely acceptable.

Whatever you choose, keep in mind that you can only exercise when you are at ease. This is necessary to ensure which you complete the workout session safely.

It is important to remember which fasted workouts aren't needed to reap the benefits of intermittent fasting. This is optional, and it is up to you to determine whether or not you want to do it.

11.8 Keep Yourself Busy During Fast

It is common to feel weird not eating when you are starting on an intermittent fasting journey. Long-term dietary habits and routines are primarily to blame. You might notice that you eat out of habit rather than need most of the time.

So, to avoid succumbing to the unwanted temptations by eating and out habit on fasting days, continue to put yourself occupied. If you do not have a job, consider picking up a hobby and keep your mind busy. To take your mind off food, read a book, call a friend, or go for a walk outside.

11.9 Take BCAAs

Intermittent fasting will cause muscle loss if you fast for long periods and miss meals. Taking BCAAs has been the only step to prevent this problem.

BCAAs (branched-chain amino acids) can be highly beneficial to people who fast intermittently. These proteins penetrate your bloodstream and aid in the development of muscle tissue.

Furthermore, BCAAs get the ability to circumvent the liver's degradation process and penetrate the bloodstream directly. As a result, they can be a perfect way to get instant energy without consuming something.

11.10 Maintain Consistency

It is not easy to begin an intermittent fasting diet. When your body adjusts to fasting, you may feel dizzy, fatigued with low blood sugar, or have other minor issues. Although these symptoms usually subside after the first week of fasting, they may be difficult to deal with. During the fasting window, you may notice yourselves slipping up and feeding. But keep in mind that it is all right.

All you have to do now is remain consistent, and you'll be fine. It requires time for the body to adjust to intermittent fasting, so make mistakes until then. Keeping a journal is one way to keep on track.

Conclusion

In conclusion, intermittent fasting will do more benefit to your body than any other diet. It will boost your metabolism, help you save time and improve your cognition too. It has also been proven to reverse the sign of aging, making you feel and look a lot younger. You can follow so many different methods and start your transformation regardless of the type of fasting you chose. Being well while you do eat is important. During fasting cycles, all of the approaches we've discussed allow you to eat little, making it much more necessary to keep hydrated. Coffee and water are mostly acceptable beverages; however, they eliminate high in carbs. If you are still adding food high in sugar and calories, it will do no good. Choosing to stay hydrated when fasting ensures you get the most from intermittent fasting.

Intermittent fasting is a weight-loss tactic that first gained attention about ten years ago. The basic principle is to eat food within a certain period. You eat very little to no food outside of that window. Fasting increases metabolism, allowing the body to break down nutrients and burn calories more effectively. This also slows down DNA decay, which happens as we get older, and speeds up DNA repair, speeding down the aging process.

Fasting also raises antioxidant levels, which can help protect cells from becoming broken down by free radicals. Fasting can also help to reduce chronic inflammation that grows as people age. Intermittent fasting, according to Corey, will help people live a healthier standard of living for a prolonged period.

Intermittent fasting advantages can be amplified if you exercise regularly. "Exercising or working out ought to be performed at the end of the fasting window to get the most benefit," Corey says. "It's critical to time the workout so that it finishes just as the feeding period is about to open."

It's critical to consult with a specialist in the area, someone who has expertise setting up these systems, before beginning an intermittent fasting regimen. "Those who do not properly set up their feeding periods with the right nutritional schedule risk losing muscle mass and not reaping the full benefits of adopting such a protocol," Corey explained.

"Intermittent fasting is a healthy and reliable weight loss, anti-aging, and overall health strategy," Corey said. "This encourages people to think about the diet they're eating and why they're eating it. It can be a beneficial initiative for a significant number of people."

This book will help you choose the best method for you and help you restrict the number of calories, but it's best to start slow as you're in your 50s, and we don't want you to put your body into a lot of stress. If your body fasting is a new concept, it will always take time to get used to it. It will be best to consult your doctor before starting intermittent fasting

Made in United States
North Haven, CT
28 October 2021